Reconstruction Surgery and Traumatology

Reconstruction Surgery
and Traumatology

Vol. 14

Condidit M. Lange, München

Editors: A. De Araujo, Rio de Janeiro; L. Böhler, Wien; J. Böhler, Wien;
E. L. Compere, Chicago, Ill.; G. Du Toit, Pretoria; E. K. Frey, München;
St. Friberg, Stockholm; F. Grospic, Zagreb; G. Hohmann, München;
F. Jimeno-Vidal, Barcelona; R. Merle d'Aubigné, Paris;
F. E. De Godoy Moreira, Sao Paulo; S. Nagura, Nagoya; R. Nissen, Basel;
C. E. Ottolenghi, Buenos Aires; H. Platt, Manchester; O. Scaglietti, Firenze;
E. Spira, Tel Aviv; W. Taillard, Genève; A. N. Witt, Berlin

Editor-in-Chief: G. Chapchal, Luzern

101 figures and 39 tables

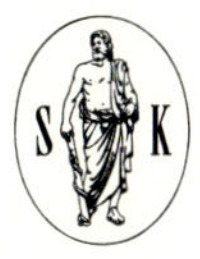

S. Karger · Basel · München · Paris · London · New York · Sydney 1974

Reconstruction Surgery and Traumatology

Vol. 1: VIII + 260 p., 101 fig., 1953. ISBN 3-8055-0606-6
Vol. 2: IV + 244 p., 319 fig., 1954.
Vol. 3: II + 181 p., 55 fig., 1956. ISBN 3-8055-0607-4
Vol. 4: IV + 222 p., 201 fig., 2 cpl., 1957. ISBN 3-8055-0608-2
Vol. 5: VIII + 300 p., 142 fig., 1960. ISBN 3-8055-0609-0
Vol. 6: IV + 139 p., 53 fig., 6 tab., 1961. ISBN 3-8055-0610-4
Vol. 7: X + 231 p., 136 fig., 2 tab., 1963. ISBN 3-8055-0611-2
Vol. 8: VIII + 253 p., 100 fig., 26 tab., 1964. ISBN 3-8055-0612-0
Vol. 9: Hand Surgery – Bone and Joint Pathology – Femoral Neck Torsion.
        VIII + 144 p., 55 fig., 6 tab., 1967. ISBN 3-8055-0613-9
Vol. 10: MORSCHER, ERWIN: Strength and Morphology of Growth Cartilage
        under Hormonal Influence of Puberty. VIII + 104 p., 35 fig., 9 tab.,
        1967. ISBN 3-8055-0614-7
Vol. 11: VI + 207 p., 108 fig., 17 tab., 1 cpl., 1969. ISBN 3-8055-0615-5
Vol. 12: X + 262 p., 117 fig., 30 tab., 3 cpl., 1971. ISBN 3-8055-1183-3
Vol. 13: IX + 209 p., 96 fig., 10 tab., 1 cpl., 1972. ISBN 3-8055-1385-2

S. Karger · Basel · München · Paris · London · New York · Sydney
Arnold-Böcklin-Strasse 25, CH-4011 Basel (Switzerland)

Contents

Fresh Fractures of the Shaft of the Humerus – Conservative or Operative Treatment? ... 65

T. Rüedi, A. Moshfegh, K. M. Pfeiffer and M. Allgöwer, Basel

Contents **VII**

Reconstr. Surg. Traumat., vol. 14, pp. 1–37 (Karger, Basel 1974)

Hip Arthrodesis with the Cobra Head Plate and Pelvic Osteotomy

R. SCHNEIDER

Contents

Introduction

Arthrodesis has remained the therapy of last resort for a painful joint since ALBERT in Vienna [1882] reported the first knee arthrodesis and

ALBEE [1908] the first five hip arthrodeses (HA). Recognition of the biomechanics and improved instrumentation have greatly increased the success of operations on bone. The safest arthrodesis is that obtained by stable internal fixation. In 1964 we developed the cobra head plate (CHP) for HA.

In this article the problems of HA are described and the results of CHP arthrodeses combined with pelvic osteotomy (PO) are compared with those of other methods used to date. The data are taken from our experience of 8 years in 112 patients. The results are mostly those of 4–8 years follow-up: the advance in alloarthroplasty in recent years is such that indications for HA have become rare. We are able to compare these results with those of 45 HA cases which we operated using other methods. We shall show that stabilization and retention of bone viability allow one to bring about healing with bone formation and bony consolidation using the CHP and PO, even in cases of severe destructive infected osteoarthropathy. This clear indication for HA is likely to remain a valid one in the future. Stable internal fixation is an effective treatment in infections, not only in infected non-unions of the extremities but also in the most difficult infected hip joint situations where none of the previously available methods lead to comparable results.

There is good clinical and experimental evidence to show that stabilization of a well vascularized pseudarthrosis leads to bony union without removal of the intervening tissue [MÜLLER et al., 1968; MÜLLER, 1961, 1964, 1971; MÜLLER and ALLGÖWER, 1958]. The situation is similar when arthrodesis of the hip joint is carried out without previous preparation of the adjacent joint surfaces. Stabilization of an arthritic non-dislocated hip with maximum care taken to project the blood supply provides better conditions for bony union than joint resection with disturbance of the nutrient blood supply.

Basically, the degree of difficulty of an arthrodesis is dependent on the magnitude of the dislocating forces which result from normal loading of the limb and on the size and state of blood supply of the contiguous bony surfaces. For this reason HA presents a particularly difficult problem.

The principles of HA with the CHP and PO are described. Duration of hospitalization, frequency of cast fixation and results in 112 cases of HA with the CHP are compared with similar data from 45 cases of HA using other methods.

*Principles of Use of the Cobra Head Plate
in Combination with Pelvic Osteotomy*

The CHP is a compression plate, that is, an internal fixation device which exerts pressure. The stabilizing effect of an internal fixation device which exerts pressure attains a maximum at that point in the bone which is furthest away from the axis of loading. The tension band effect increases in proportion to the distance from the axis of loading, i. e. the interfragmentary pressure and with it the stabilizing interfragmentary friction rise in proportion to the load. Adequate support on the medial side is a prerequisite. The CHP lies on the lateral aspect of the pelvis and femur at a maximum distance from the axis of loading. Thus when weight is placed on the leg, maximum stabilization of the arthrodesis is obtained. Again, the plate lies as far as possible from the axis of rotation and is thus in an optimal position for prevention of rotation. Internal fixation devices which lie in the femoral neck close to the axis of rotation do not have this advantage. Prevention of flexion-extension is more difficult than achievement of rotational stability. A considerable flexion loading of the hip occurs unavoidably in the sitting position. A plate applied posteriorly would have a tension band effect and convert the bending moment at the hip joint into pressure. However, application of a plate posteriorly is excluded for anatomical reasons.

The problem of stabilization in the sagittal plane can be analyzed as follows: pelvic anchorage points must be chosen which lie as far as possible from the transverse axis of rotation. A lateral plate which is extended superiorly in a direction away from the transverse axis of rotation comes to lie over the thinner and weaker bone of the gluteal surface of the ileum. The strength of the bone in this area is normally insufficient for plate anchorage. Anteriorly and posteriorly in the region of the acetabular roof, plate anchorage points can be found which are sufficiently far from the transverse axis of rotation such that a stabilizing effect is obtained. At the same time the bone in which the anchorage screws lie is the densest of the whole pelvis. This is the reason for the transverse extension of the straight lateral plate. The original CHP was fixed in the pelvis with six screws, the upper two of which lay in the weak bone of the gluteal surface of the ileum. The plate was later shortened and of the six pelvic screws, five are fixed in dense bone.

Implants placed in the steeply angled femoral neck of a coxa valga may be deeply imbedded in the acetabular roof and thus produce sufficient fixation in the sagittal plane. In coxa vara, however, the axis of the implant approximates to the transverse axis of rotation and in addition to this it lies in the thinner pelvic bone at the acetabular base. Such implants are thus inadequate in coxa vara.

The CHP produces maximum stabilization for the reasons shown. It neutralizes the dislocating forces whatever the pre-operative anatomy.

The plate is curved in the coronal plane so as to adapt to the local anatomy. A degree of curvature is chosen such that the femur is normally medialized. The medialization is more marked and more necessary in coxa vara and less marked and less necessary in coxa valga. It leads to a reduction of the dislocating forces. It can only be produced by transverse PO at the level of the acetabular roof, with medial displacement of the distal pelvic component and slight angulation of the symphysis. The force exerted on the femur to produce medialization partially compensates for the torsion exerted during plate tensioning which tends to abduct the leg. The variable displacement allowed by PO permits one to adapt the CHP to almost any anatomical situation including coxa valga, coxa vara, a long femoral neck or a short femoral neck. Only in rare cases of coxa vara combined with a very long femoral neck is the required degree of displacement so great that the head of the femur and the distal pelvis are no longer supported medially by the ileum. This compromises the tension band effect of the CHP and the system loses its stability. *The most important advantage of PO is, however, the decisive enlargement of the area of contact between the femur and the pelvis.* In coxa valga subluxans the displacement leads to good coverage of the frequently small head by the ileum. In every case a space remains between the lateral acetabular roof, the neck of the femur and the plate. This space varies in size and can be filled with a trochanteric graft which produces a welcome increase in the size of the bony bridge between the pelvis and the femur. This graft which is under pressure, and therefore in a stable situation, becomes rapidly incorporated. The area of bone contact is not only increased but also remains free of implant material. This can be important in cases of infection. The head of the femur is not dislocated during CHP arthrodesis and there is less damage to the blood supply than in methods which involve dislocation and preparation of the opposing surfaces. The CHP arthrodesis with PO produces maximum stability, increases the areas of contact across which bony union takes place, protects the blood supplies of these areas and thereby brings about suitable conditions for rapid bone healing. The procedure allows one to choose the degree of flexion or

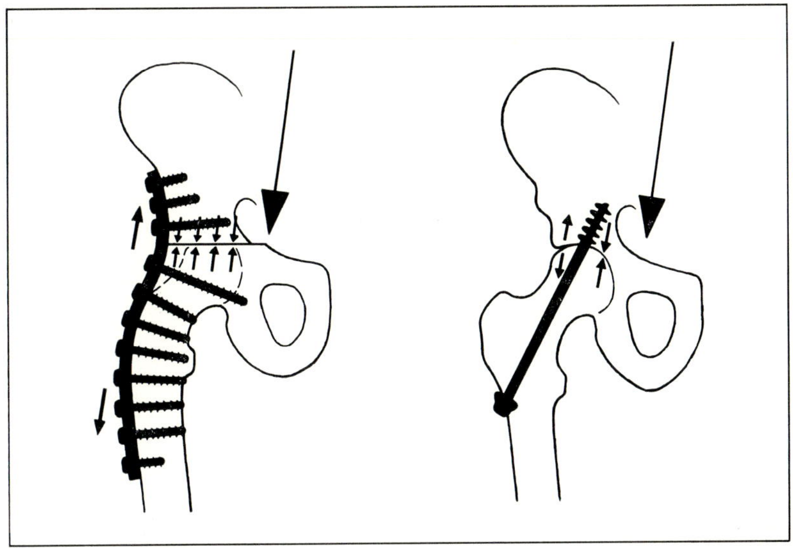

Fig. 1. Left: Tension band effect of the CHP on loading the leg. The pressure produced gives rise to interfragmentary friction over the full extent of the opposing surfaces. The bone graft which is introduced laterally is fixed under pressure. The healing bone surface is large and free from internal fixation material. The joint is not dislocated and there is therefore maximum preservation of the nutrient blood supply of the femoral head. Right: In any fixation using a femoral neck implant (nail, screw, compression nail), loading lateral to the implant tends to distract the fragments. This reduces or abolishes the stabilizing friction. An ileofemoral graft is never under pressure and is therefore only loosely held in place. The healing bone surface is smaller and is additionally reduced by an amount equal to the cross-sectional area of the implant.

extension in each case to suit the individual functional requirements of the patient. A post-operative cast is normally not applied. In severe osteoporosis, or in the presence of osteolysis accompanying bone-joint infections, the pelvic screw fixation is insufficiently solid to allow omission of a post-operative cast. A hip spica has to be applied to protect the stable but nevertheless vulnerable fixation from forces which would tend to cause dislocation. If the hip spica is omitted in these cases there is usually bone formation but, because of the instability, absence of bony union. Reoperation and restabilization of the CHP fixation usually brings about rapid healing. The absence of a cast simplifies the post-operative management and mobilisation of the joint. We have never observed significant limitation of knee joint movement.

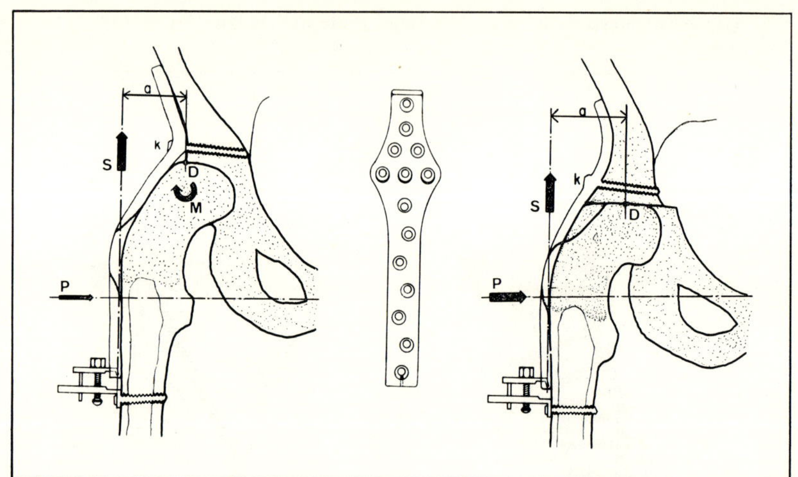

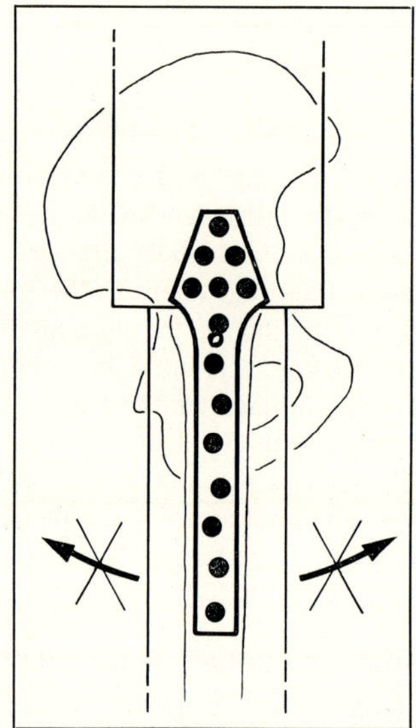

Fig. 2. Compensation for torque produced during plate tensioning by the increased opposing pressure of the CHP generated by displacement of the PO. (a) Torque ($M = S. a$) is produced during tightening of the tensioning device. Frequently the fixation of the plate to the pelvis is inadequate to withstand this torque and the leg goes into abduction. (b) The force P is produced by tightening the screw k. This displaces the femur medially together with the pelvis. On tensioning the plate a torque $= S. a$ is produced about the axis of rotation D. Experience has shown however that this torque is compensated for by the force P. The leg remains in equilibrium.

Fig. 3. Stabilization produced by the CHP in the sagittal plane. The transverse axis of rotation passes between the two upper femoral screws.

KALÉN [1968] used an anatomical preparation to compare the stability of the CHP with that of staggered nails. He found the nail fixation to be more stable. However, the CHP in his model was not fixed in the dense iliac bone of the acetabular roof but rather too high on the thin gluteal surface of the thin blade of the ileum. In addition, the surface of contact had not been increased by PO. The CHP is a tension band device and the test of abduction stability which was carried out can be compared to the exertion of pressure on the arch of a bridge from underneath.

The Ideal Post-Arthrodesis Hip Joint Position

We aimed for a neutral position between adduction and abduction, flexion of 150–160° and external rotation of 10°. If the opposite side is normal, a position should be chosen which results in 1 cm of leg shortening. We use an ordinary operating table and comparison of leg length by placing the feet together and palpating the medial malleolae is therefore simple. The reader is referred to the work of LINDAHL [1965] on the connection between adduction and leg length. The degree of flexion depends on the position of the patient, body weight, and the condition of the vertebral column and of the opposite hip joint. MERLE D'AUBIGNÉ et al. [1964] and AHLBÄCK and LINDAHL [1966] have given us very instructive directions on this subject. BOUILLET and DELCHEF [1968] and MERLE D'AUBIGNÉ et al. [1964] warn of the unphysiological valgus loading of the knee joint produced by excessive abduction and BOUILLET and DELCHEF consider excessive internal rotation to be a cause of osteoarthritis of the knee joint. The angle of adduction can be measured during the operation using the Müller coxometer and the angles of adduction and flexion can be measured using the two-plane protractor developed by FICHTNER [1969]. The degree of pelvic tilt, i. e. of lumbar lordosis, must be known if the degree of flexion is to be measured accurately. If severe lumbar lordosis is present, the hip has usually to be fused with the leg in maximum extension.

Indication

The success of the total hip prosthesis operation in recent years has led to a marked reduction in the number of indications for HA. Today

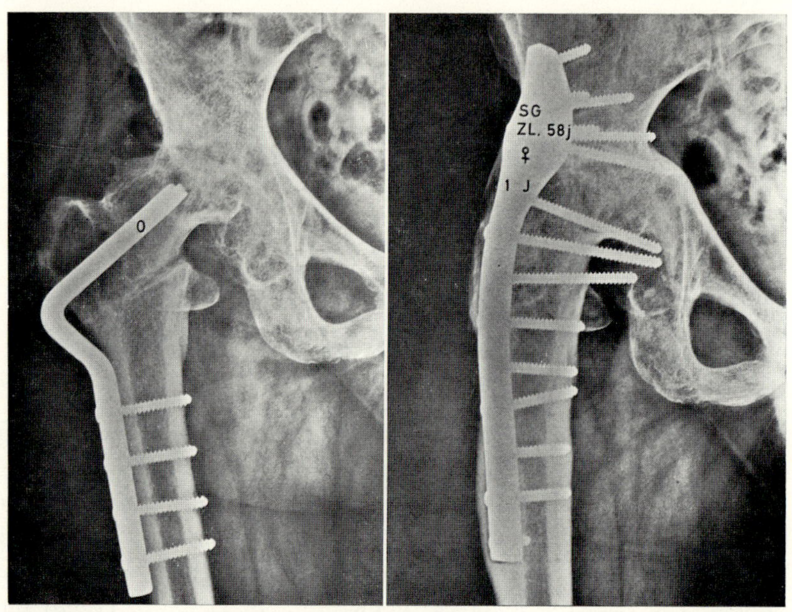

4

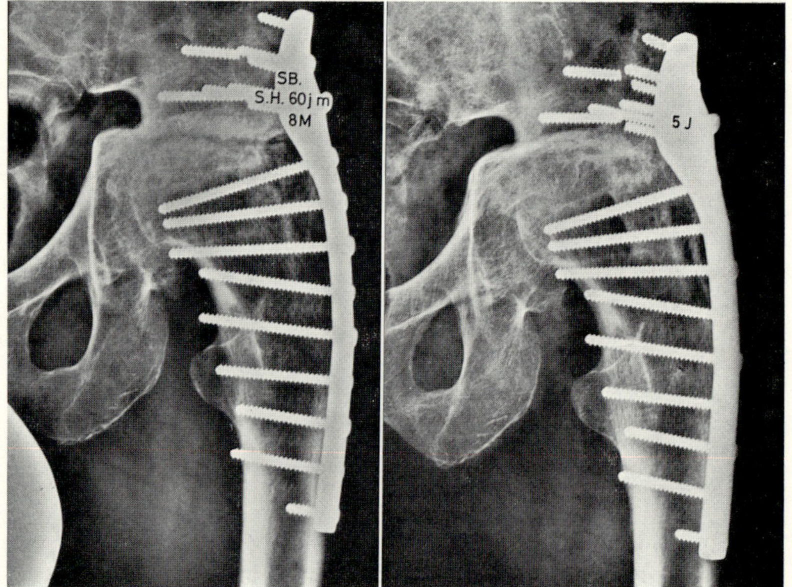

5

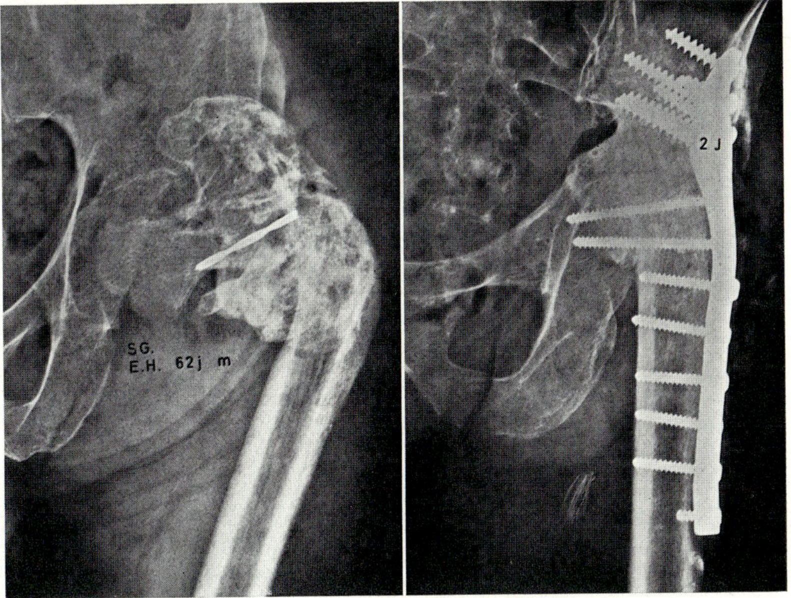

Fig. 4. Status following unsatisfactory intertrochanteric osteotomy with lateral subluxation of a small head in a housekeeper aged 57 years. The increase in area of the uniting bony surfaces using the CHP in combination with PO is demonstrated.

Fig. 5. Farmer aged 60 years. Instability led to fracture of the pelvic screws. There was no union at 8 months but the patient was still able to work. Spontaneous union occured without further treatment. Despite the lucky outcome, this case demonstrates that medialization and a large area of contact predispose to bony consolidation.

Fig. 6. Severely alcoholic carpenter, aged 62 years. Status following internal fixation of a pertrochanteric fracture. Staphylococcal infection of bone and joint with fistula and osteolysis in the acetabular roof. Bony union following stabilization with CHP and PO and post-operative hip spica.

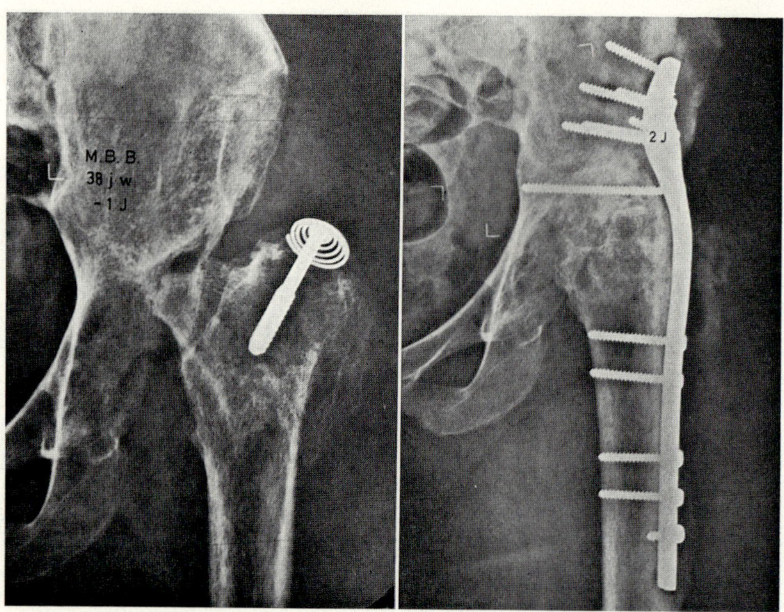

7

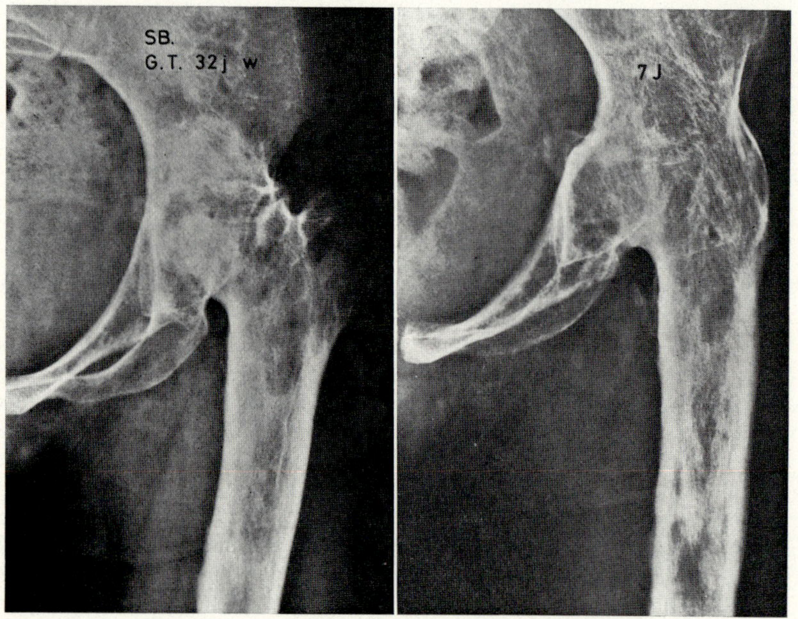

8

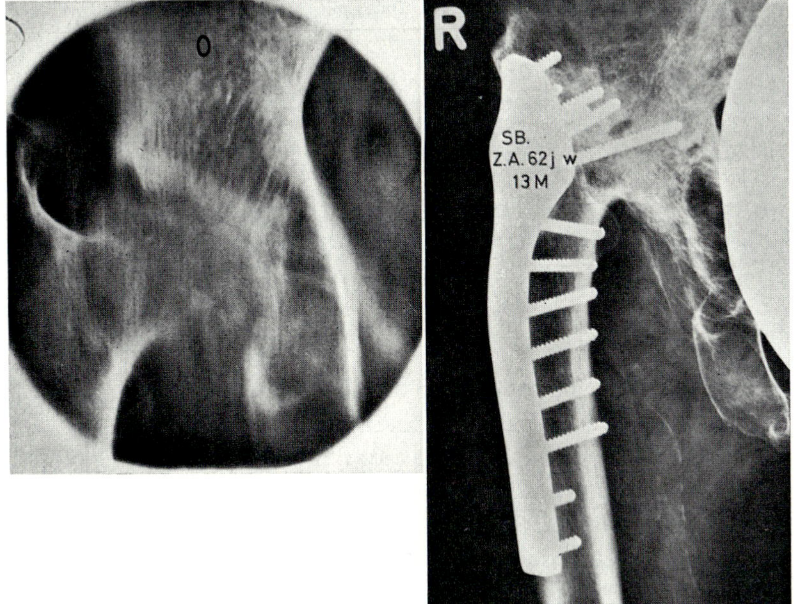

9

Fig. 7. Obese nursing sister, aged 38 years, with destructive fistulous tuberculitic hip and superimposed staphylococcal infection. Status following drilling of the femoral neck, arthrodesis, opening of the abcess and sequestrotomy. The patient had been bedridden and incapable of walking for 2½ years. Osteoporosis. Refusal of a post-operative hip spica. Bone regeneration and union following reoperation with hip spica. Normal pain-free weight bearing is possible and the patient has recovered her full working capacity. The fairly stiff knee joint was submitted to the full Judet operation. The active range of movement is 175–100°; passive movement up to 80°.

Fig. 8. Businesswoman aged 33 years. Painful fistulous haematogenic staphylococcal infection of bone and joint in the left hip, which commenced at age 12 years. Healed following CHP arthrodesis with PO. Removal of the plate one year later. Subsequently completely complaint-free with good scar.

Fig. 9. Farmer's wife aged 61 years with destructive tuberculosis of the hip. Solid bony union 13 months following arthrodesis with CHP and PO and reoperation with hip spica.

Indications in 157 Arthrodeses of the Hip

Osteoarthritis of the hip	145
Tuberculosis of the hip joint	4
Tuberculosis plus staphylococcal infection	2
Staphylococcal infection of bone and joint	2
Osteoarthritis with femoral neck fracture	2
Osteoarthritis with subtrochanteric femoral fracture	1
Head necrosis following femoral neck fracture	1

the most suitable indications for arthrodesis of the hip are bacterial infections of bone and joint or osteoarthritis in young patients in whom an osteotomy seems to be inapplicable or has failed. The healing of fistulous staphylococcal infections of the hip joint following arthrodesis with the CHP and PO proves the effectiveness of stable internal fixation as a therapy against infection. The same is of course true for tuberculosis. In motor paralysis or other cases of severe muscular insufficiency the rigidity of a stiffened hip joint is frequently of more help to the patient than, for example, a total prosthesis [CENNI, 1966; HANSLIK and FRIEDEBOLD, 1970]. HA is particularly suitable for small patients and for those who must carry out heavy manual work, as long as the other joints and the vertebral column are not affected. It should be pointed out here that a patient who has already become used to a marked degree of joint stiffness and simply wishes to be relieved of pain is a much more suitable candidate for HA than one whose hip joint is still freely mobile. The degree of hinderance of daily activity produced by an arthrodesis increases markedly with body height. A patient with a fixed hip has relatively little difficulty in sitting on a high chair but a low chair presents considerable problems. A chair of normal height is relatively high for the small patient and relatively low for the large patient. I therefore include body height as one of the important criteria in deciding whether an arthrodesis is indicated or not. Surprisingly, I can find no reference to this factor in the literature.

Arthrodesis of one hip was combined with total prosthesis, intertrochanteric osteotomy or Girdlestone operation of the opposite hip in 45 cases of bilateral osteoarthritis on the principle that the freely movable hip would be relieved of load by the fixed weight-bearing leg on the opposite side. The cases were distributed as follows:

CHP and PO combined with total prosthesis	20
Other arthrodeses combined with total prosthesis	9
CHP combined with intertrochanteric osteotomy	5
Other arthrodeses combined with intertrochanteric osteotomy	8
CHP combined with Girdlestone	1
Other arthrodeses combined with Girdlestone	2

*Technique of Hip Arthrodesis with Pelvic Osteotomy
and Cobra Head Plate*

The patient is placed supine on a conventional operating table. The leg which is to be operated is covered by a large transparent plastic film which extends from the umbilicus down to the lower leg. In addition it covers the genital area and the opposite leg as far as the middle of the thigh. The drapes are applied in such a manner that the leg which is to be operated is freely movable. Its position can easily be visually checked during the operation. Both medial malleoli must be easily palpable so that the functional leg length can be compared during the operation. If marked flexion contracture is not present a rolled towel is placed under the knee joint so as to bring the leg into the required flexion position. The lateral incision commences 3–4 fingerbreadths cranial to the tip of the greater trochanter and runs 25–30 cm distally. The iliotibial tract is split and the upper component of the vastus lateralis muscle is freed from the innominate line and from the intermuscular septum. The vastus lateralis is retracted anteromedially with Hohmann retractors. All the trochanteric muscle insertions are removed by decortication with an osteotome. The joint capsule is exposed using Hohmann retractors and the anterior and superior part is excised. Following excision of the capsule, the gluteus medius and gluteus minimus muscles can be lifted away laterally using a Hohmann retractor which is driven in high up in the blade of the ileum. Thus good exposure of the lateral aspect of the pelvis superior to the hip joint is produced. In addition, Hohmann retractors which lie close to the bone are driven anteriorly and posteriorly into the pelvis. Using scalpel, rasp and osteotome, the joint line is exposed laterally and the area of bone which will lie under the plate is smoothed off. If the blade of the ileum is markedly curved or if the pelvis is small, the plate will not lie flat on the bone. In such cases the plate must be sunk in a depression which is cut out anteriorly with the osteotome. The plate is thus directed somewhat posteriorly, which is not disadvantageous. Fears that this countersinking of the plate may shorten the distance within which the screws lie in bone and thereby weaken their hold, are groundless. On the contrary, the more posterior direction of the screws lengthens their path in bone and particularly their path through the internal cortex, through which they pass obliquely. The net result is a significant improvement of the screw hold.

A bone surface is prepared by cutting away the greater trochanter and the cranial surface of the femoral neck with the oscillating saw. The transverse PO passes in a medial direction at the level of the upper border of the hip joint and is carried out as far as possible with the oscillating saw. It is completed with a flat osteotome shielded by Hohmann retractors. It is important that this osteotome should not be allowed to jam in the osteotomy since this severely reduces the surgeon's ability to judge the extent of the cut. Jamming is prevented by inserting a wedge-shaped osteotome or spreading forceps into the osteotomy. On completion of the pelvic osteotomy it is relatively easy to displace the distal part of the pelvis medially together with the femur using a broad osteotome. A flat cranial segment of the head of the femur is usually sliced off when a PO is carried out with the oscillating saw. This flat segment is removed. The angles of flexion, adduction and rotation of the leg are checked. The CHP is applied. It should lie parallel to the shaft of the femur and is bent if necessary. The position of the central hole in the CHP is determined; it should be approximately 5 mm above the joint line in the acetabular roof and parallel to the PO. The hole is drilled, the thread is cut and the bone thickness is measured. The central screw is inserted. Tightening of this screw causes the femur and the distal pelvis to be pushed medially by the plate, and the resulting pelvic displacement improves the coverage of the head and of the superior aspect of the femoral neck. At this point there is a danger that the screw be overloaded and lose its hold. The displacement is therefore carried out stepwise, using a bent osteotome which is inserted into the osteotomy and used as a lever. This allows the screw to be easily tightened without overloading. The plate is fixed to the shaft of the femur with Verbrugge clamps. The plate tensioner is applied, the osteotomy is provisionally placed under pressure, and the position of the leg is checked. If the latter is correct, the remaining screws are inserted in the head of the

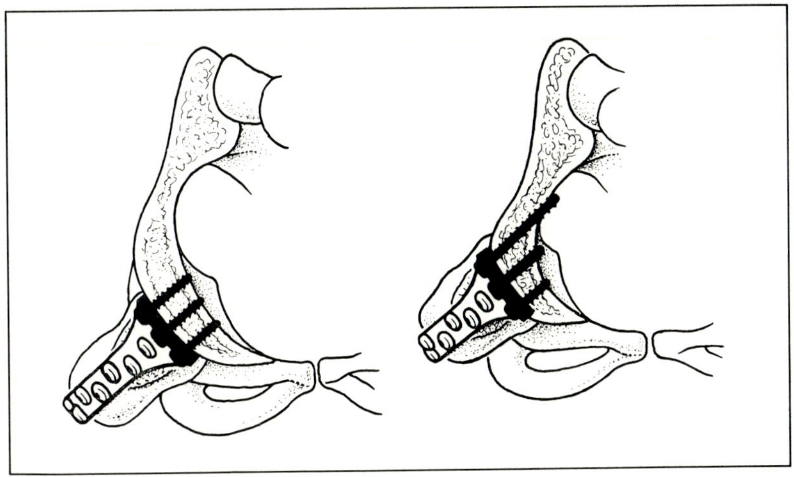

Fig. 10. If the CHP does not lie flat on the bone, a recess is cut for it anteriorly in the ileum with the osteotome. This increases the posterior inclination of the plate which in turn lengthens the path of the screws in bone and causes them to pass obliquely through the internal cortex.

plate. Additional bending of the CHP is unnecessary in the majority of cases. Correction of the leg position is only possible by removing the plate and bending it. At this point palpation of the medial malleoli should be carried out in addition to the visual check. The operated leg should usually be 1 cm shorter. As a rule, in coxa vara a small groove is cut at the level of the innominate line into which the plate is recessed. The trochanteric fragment which is to be inserted into the triangular space between the lateral aspect of the acetabular roof, the prepared surface of the femoral neck, and the plate, is cut to size. Additional cortico-cancellous chips are inserted anteriorly, posteriorly and laterally between the head and the acetabular roof. The plate tensioner is now tightened, producing strong compression between the head, the pelvis, the bone chips and the plate. The result is a stable internal fixation which has the mechanical properties of a tension band. The remaining screws are inserted with exact measurement of the screw length. The upper two screws immediately adjacent to the head of the plate are usually 70 mm long cortex screws. These obtain a hold in and fix the distal pelvic component. The most distal screw is a 16-mm cortex screw which only passes through 1 cortex. This renders the change in elasticity between the plate and the distal bone less abrupt and reduces the danger of fracture following relatively mild trauma; we have found this danger to be most marked in the first postoperative

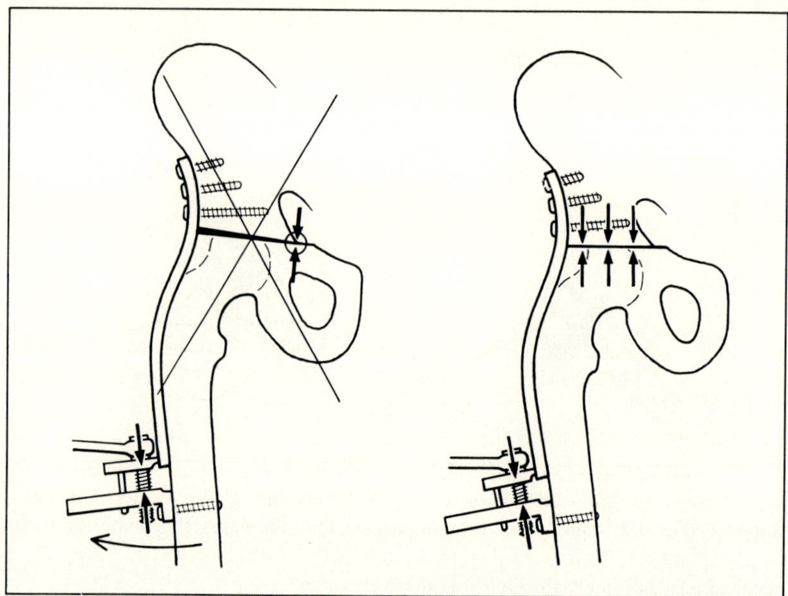

Fig. 11. The PO must lie in the horizontal plane. If it slopes distally, medial displacement results in leg lengthening and formation of a medial pivot. The pivot effect arises as a result of the greater solidity of the medial support when compared to the lateral support produced by the trochanteric graft. In such cases the CHP pulls the leg into excessive abduction.

months. The wound is closed in layers with careful suturing together of the abductors and the vastus lateralis over the plate. Two Redivac drains are put in place for 48 h. The average blood requirement is 1.5 l of whole blood. We do not apply a post-operative cast if the screw fixation is adequate. If the hold of the screws in the bone is inadequate because of osteolytic processes, a hip spica is applied for 3 months either immediately post-operatively or before the patient gets out of bed. The patient gets up with partial weight bearing after 2–3 weeks; he must be able to lift the extended leg without pain before this is allowed (fig. 10).

Technical Errors

The plane of the PO must be horizontal. If it slopes caudally medial displacement leads to leg lengthening and formation of an extreme medial

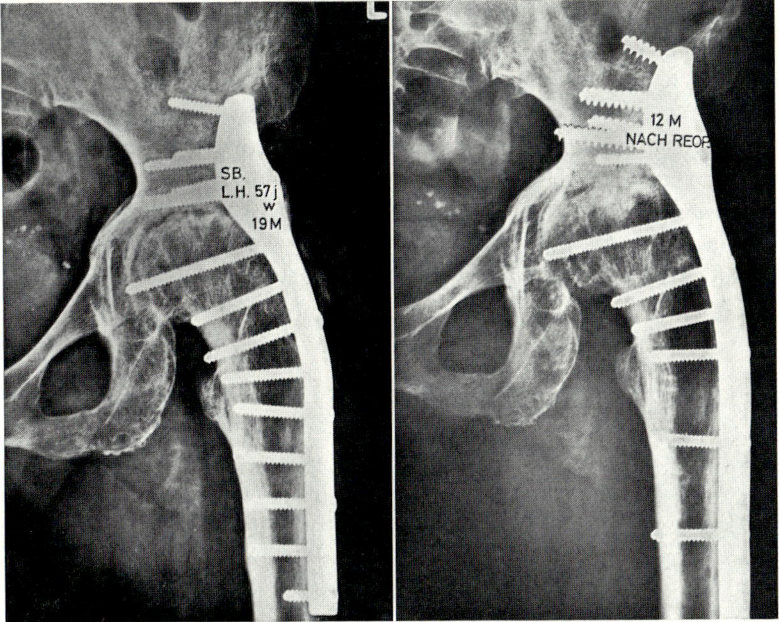

Fig. 12. Housewife aged 55 years. Instability with unsure gait and mild pain 19 months following CHP arthrodesis and PO. Reoperation with replacement of the pelvic cortex screws by cancellous screws and use of a longer plate with less screws in the femur (the number of screws used is kept proportional to the degree of implant reinforcement actually required by the bone). Bony union following reoperation.

pivot. In this situation, application of compression with the plate tensioning device leads to abduction deformity as described by DREYER and PINGEL [1969].

The plate should on no account be fastened to the flat thin bone of the blade of the ilium since the fixation at this point is inadequate. The lowest screw of the pelvic fixation should lie in the sclerotic bone of the acetabular roof approximately 5 mm above the PO.

In cases of coxa vara with a long femoral neck, excessive medial displacement causes the head to lose its support against the ilium. This leads to a significant loss of stability. In these cases we supplement the fixation with a hip spica for 8–10 weeks or reduce the displacement by medial head resection.

The CHP provides less stable fixation of a Charnley arthrodesis [DE MONTMOLLIN, 1968], because of the inadequate medial support. In addition there is a marked loss of leg length.

Chisel blows to the femur can cause fissuring and lead later to fatigue fractures. They should be avoided at all costs. The trochanter should be removed with the oscillating saw.

In cases where the bone is osteoporotic, a condition which is frequently met in connection with destructive bone pathology of infectious origin, the stable but nevertheless vulnerable fixation should be protected against overloading by application of a hip spica. If for some reason this additional external support cannot be used, the possible failure of bony union should be borne in mind and the necessity for reoperation with a new CHP should be anticipated (fig. 11).

Technique of Reoperation for Instability

In cases where failure of bony union gives rise to symptoms of clinical significance, reoperation almost always results in final consolidation. The unstable zone contains well vascularized, resistant, mostly dense bone which usually reacts to restabilization by rapidly uniting the bony fragments. The plate is exposed and removed using the same approach. The bone surface which lay in contact with the plate is cleaned up. The unstable zone becomes immediately apparent on moving the leg. Now all that is necessary is to replace the old plate with a new one which is longer by 2 screw holes. It is important that the old fatigued plate be discarded. In two cases the old plate was even fractured. The simplest procedure is to implant the new plate at the site of the old one. The unstable 4.5 mm cortex screws which lie in the pelvis become surrounded by sclerotic bone and are usually best replaced by 6.5 mm cancellous screws of 32 mm length which usually obtain a good hold. Another method which can be used to firmly anchor the new plate in the pelvis is that based on the 'swinging hole mechanism'. Using the same hole of entry, a second screw hole is drilled at an angle of 15 to 30° to the old one. Because the screw hole is longer it is best drilled in a posterior direction. Fragments of broken screws should be left *in situ,* since their removal would excessively weaken the bone in which the plate is fixed. There is sufficient stability for cast-free post-operative management if 5–6 screws have a firm hold. In the femoral shaft, a possible change in leg position and the retensioning of the fixation allows one to find sufficient hold in solid bone. Here, too, the 'swinging hole mechanism' can be used to implant a screw in more solid bone in the opposite

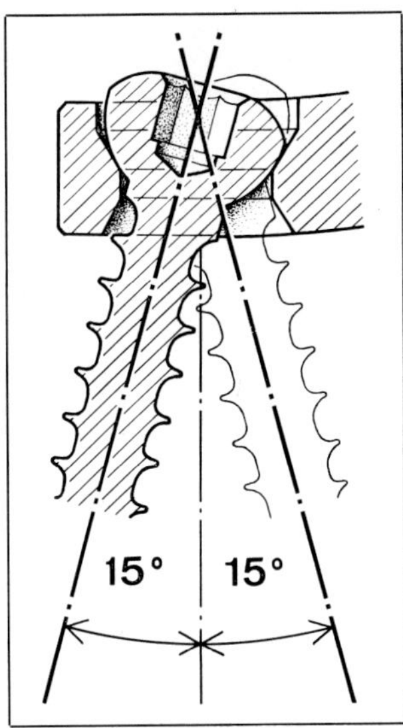

Fig. 13. The 'swinging hole mechanism' involves angular displacement of the screw at reoperation, thus giving it a better hold in new bone.

cortex. Only rigidly sited screws should be left in place. As in the pelvis, fragments of broken screws should be left in place. The use of a plate which is 2 holes longer than the old one increases the plate fixation by 3 cortices and the femoral plate fixation at reoperation is therefore simple. During reoperation for instability it is possible to correct any mal-positioning of the leg (almost always an adduction deformity) in the unstable zone or, exceptionally, by intertrochanteric osteotomy with removal of a small lateral bone wedge. Slight bending of the new plate may be necessary to make it fit the new hip angle (fig. 12, 13).

Technique in Fixed Deformity

Deformity with bony union following CHP arthrodesis is rare. The plate is removed and the deformity is corrected by intertrochanteric osteotomy and removal of an appropriate bone wedge. The osteotomy must be carried out with the oscillating saw and is fixed under compression, either with a CHP or with a straight broad plate which has been suitably bent (fig. 14).

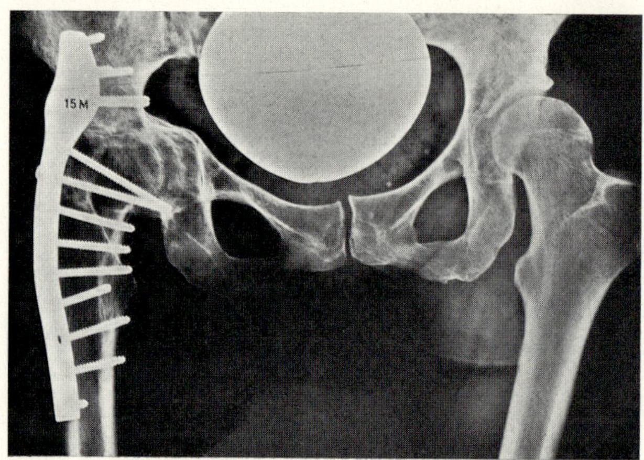

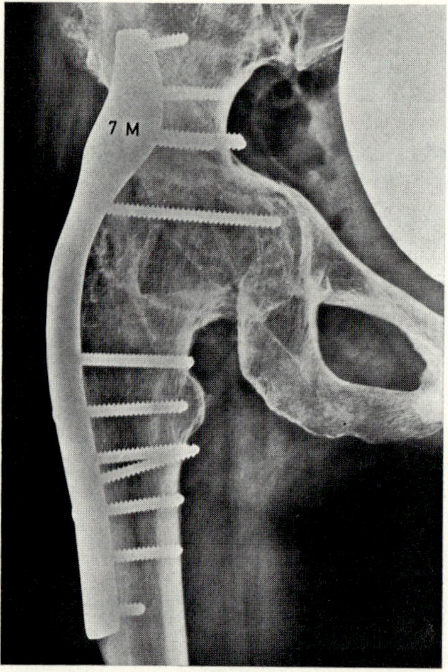

Fig. 14. Housewife aged 40 years. Abduction deformity with 2 cm increase in functional leg length. Technique of corrective osteotomy. A transverse cut is made as high up as possible and a medial wedge is removed. Rigid fixation is obtained using a markedly bent CHP. Rapid union. Reduction in leg length of 0.5 cm; 3° adduction.

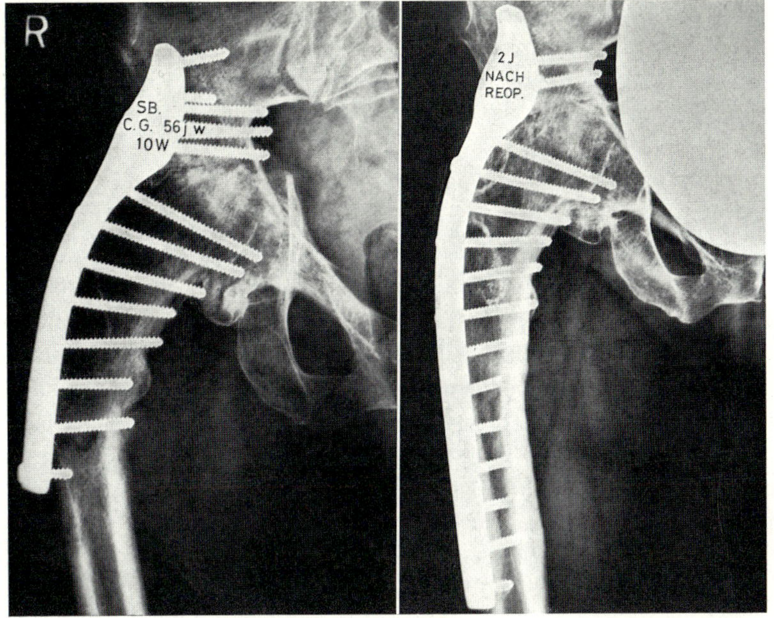

Fig. 15. Housewife aged 56 years. Femoral fracture following trivial trauma. 10 weeks following operation and 5 weeks after discharge from hospital. Technique of reoperation using longer CHP. Rapid union. No cast. The patient got up and commenced partial weight bearing 4 weeks post-operatively.

Technique in Cases of Femoral Fracture
at the Distal End of the Plate

Until bony union has occurred with adaptation of the skeleton to the new static and dynamic circumstances, there is a danger of fracture at the lower end of the plate following relatively insignificant trauma. These fractures are usually short and oblique, and occur as a result of the difference in elasticity between the plate and the bone distal to it. Anatomical reduction is easy and the fracture is fixed with a new CHP which is 5–6 holes longer than the one which it replaces. Thus the screws in the distal fragment have a hold in 9 cortices, which allows cast-free post-operative management despite the considerable leverage of the leg.

These fractures usually heal rapidly since bone turnover in the area in question is considerably increased and with it the activity of the Haversian system. The patient can get out of bed with partial weight bearing after 4 weeks! As in all internal fixations, moderation is called for in the fixation of fractures at the lower end of the plate and it is unnecessary to place screws in all the proximal holes (fig. 15).

The Question of Plate Removal

Removal of the CHP was carried out in only 2 out of the 108 CHP arthrodeses which we carried out mainly between 1965 and 1968. In one case an infection was present and in the other case there was pain in the region of the implant. Basically, at least one year should be allowed to elapse before a CHP is removed in order that one can be sure of adequate bony union. It should be remembered that the femoral bone which lies under the plate remains weak for several months following plate removal and there should therefore be adequate protection from overloading during this period. However, analysis of our series of CHPs to date shows the bone implant to be well tolerated.

Results and Complications
of Cobra Head Plate Arthrodesis with Pelvic Osteotomy Compared
to Other Hip Arthrodesis Techniques

The CHP was used in 112 patients between 1965 and 1970: 83 patients were operated in the Grosshöchstetten District Hospital and 29 in other clinics. Four patients died post-operatively and 1 patient could not be followed up so that 107 cases remain for analysis. These 107 CHP arthrodeses can be compared with 45 HAs which were carried out between 1960 and 1968 using other methods.

We have full data on the indications, radiological results, subjective results and complications from the 107 cases of arthrodesis.

In addition, we have data on the localization of pre- and post-operative pain in a group of 48 patients from the Grosshöchstetten District Hospital in whom a CHP arthrodesis was carried out between 12. 1. 1965 and 1. 10. 1966. For the purposes of analysis the localization of the pain was divided into back, iliosacrum, symphysis, upper leg and knee. Mobility, capacity for work, weight, height, actual and functional leg length, angle of abduction and adduction measured with the coxometer, pre-operative flexion, extension, range of rotation, neutral rotation position and duration of hospital stay were all measured. The data thus obtained from this group can be considered as representative of the whole group of 107 cases of CHP arthrodesis.

Follow-up was possible in all 42 cases from the Grosshöchstetten District Hospital in which arthrodesis was carried out using other methods. We have full information on indication, technique, complications, subjective results, radiological results and duration of hospital stay in these cases.

Other Arthrodesis Techniques

Key grafting with intertrochanteric osteotomy, cast	22
Key grafting without intertrochanteric osteotomy, cast	9
Straight plate, PO, graft, cast	8
Long straight plate, graft, cast	2
Charnley, cast	2
Double nail (completion of spontaneous but not quite complete healing in a large head), without cast	1
Screw fixation, cast	1

It should be noted here that the 8 cases which were treated with a plate and PO belong in principle to the group treated with CHP arthrodesis and PO. They were the forerunners of the modern technique.

Comparison of Results

	CHP with pelvic osteotomy, n = 107	Other arthrodeses, n = 45
Stable bony union following the first operation	94 (88)	40 (89)
Stable bony union following reoperation	6 (5.5)	5 (11)
No bony union, no reoperation	7 (6.5)	0 (0)
Post-operative cast	11 (10)	44 (97)
Average range of knee movement, degrees	178–57	176–77
Duration of hospital stay, days	44	80

Percentages given in parentheses.

In comparing the two groups of arthrodeses it should be noted that the indication in the CHP arthrodesis group on grounds of cast-free post-operative management and early mobilization was also extended to patients in whom extensive immobilization was excluded because of their age or general condition. In addition, cases of destructive bacterial osteoarthropathy were operated using the CHP. These difficult starting conditions should be borne in mind when interpreting the instability and re-operation rate in this group. On the other hand, the comparison between the groups is rendered more valid by the fact that the earlier arthrodeses were all carried out by the chief surgeon, while only a part of the CHP group of patients was operated by the senior resident.

Investigation of a group of 50 CHP arthrodeses was carried out with 3 follow-ups at an average of 18 months following operation. In particular, the patients were questioned about pain caused by the PO and the resulting distortion at the symphysis and sacroiliac joints. In addition, we were particularly interested in the position of the leg following CHP arthrodesis. The stress on the vertebral column is increased and the question of back pain and its dependence on weight and height had to be clarified.

Preoperative status: All patients complained of severe hip pain which radiated from the trochanter or the groin to the upper leg and knee.

14 patients complained specifically of accompanying back pain. Severe pain over the sacroiliac joint or pain over the symphysis was not reported. The walking distance (with or without the aid of sticks) lay between 5 m and 5 km, the average being 1.3 km.

Functional leg length between +2.0 and −6.0 cm (mean: −2.2 cm)
Range of flexion between 0 and 70° (mean: 24°)
Extension between 125 and 180° (mean: 157°)
Range of rotation between 0 (30 cases) and 40°
Midpoint between extreme internal rotation and extreme external rotation lay between 20 and 40°, respectively.
Weight between 48 and 95 kg (mean: 69.5 kg)
Height between 140 and 175 cm (mean: 162 cm)

Post-operative status at 15 months: 48 cases; 2 post-operative deaths.

Subjective findings: all patients had few complaints and were satisfied with the result. Freedom from hip pain and improved mobility were mentioned by the patients as being the chief benefits of the operation. Difficulty in tying shoelaces and in sitting down and, frequently, unsure gait on uneven ground were described as disadvantages.

Back pain: The following results were obtained in 14 patients with preexisting lumbar pain:

Reduction of pain	6
Unchanged	6
Worsened	2

6 patients who had had no pre-operative back pain mentioned it as a post-operative symptom

Sacroiliac Pain

Slight pain, sensitivity to weather	7
Pain in the symphyseal region	0
Slight pain in the groin and thigh	9
Pain in knee	5

Height, weight, age and walking distance of patients who complained of pain: The mean weight was 74 kg which was 5 kg greater than the mean weight of all the patients taken together. The mean height was 168 cm which was 6 cm greater than the mean of the whole group. The mean age of 61 years was identical with that of all the patients taken together. The mean walking distance was 3.2 km. Functional leg length – 1.9 cm. Mean distance from anterior superior iliac spine to medial malleolus – 1.2 cm.

Adduction angle: 50 %, 86–88°; 50 %, 78–94°. Extension angle: 60 %, 155–160°; 40 %, 135–165°.

Midpoint between extreme internal rotation and extreme external rotation lay between 5 and 40°, respectively (mean was 17° external rotation). Mean range of knee movement, 178–57°.

It can be seen from this group of cases that failure of bony union following CHP arthrodesis does not necessarily cause severe problems. Instability following other techniques caused more problems. All the cases had to be reoperated.

Reoperation in Cases of Instability

Six cases of CHP arthrodesis

Head necrosis following femoral neck fracture. Union following second CHP arthrodesis without cast ... 1

Mixed tuberculitic infection. Union following second CHP arthrodesis and hip spica ... 1

Osteoarthritis of the hip. Healing following second CHP without cast ... 4

Five cases using other techniques

Tuberculosis. Arthrodesis with graft, straight plate and cast. Union with CHP and cast ... 1

Osteoarthritis of the hip. Screw fixation with key grafting. Union following intertrochanteric osteotomy and condylar plate with cast ... 1

Osteoarthritis with graft and intertrochanteric osteotomy. Union following condylar plate in 2 cases and double nail in 1 case. All with cast ... 3

Seven cases without bony union following the first CHP arthrodesis

Stable, almost completely complaint-free, satisfied and 100 % fit for work as farmer and butcher. Could not be persuaded to undergo reoperation ... 2

Satisfied, almost complaint-free, retired ... 2

Psychiatrist aged 61 years with high congenital dislocation and very thin pelvis who refused the necessary post-operative cast because of claustrophobia acquired during the Messina earthquake. Insecure stance $3^1/_4$ years following operation but allegedly pain-free and satisfied ... 1

Widow aged 71 years. The only infected arthrodesis with osteomyelitis. Plate removal and wound perfusion was followed by healing of the infection. New joint formation occurred after 5 years. The patient, who resides in a home for old people, is satisfied and refuses reoperation ... 1

Master gardener aged 60 years. Severe bilateral osteoarthritis of the hip joint. Bilateral intertrochanteric osteotomy performed. Considerable instability following left-sided CHP arthrodesis. Plate fracture. Right-sided total prosthesis 5 years later and conversion of the left-sided arthrodesis into a total prosthesis ... 1

Reoperation in Cases of Malposition

	CHP arthrodesis (n = 108)	Other techniques (n = 45)
Abduction malposition	2	0
Adduction malposition	1	2 (following IO with graft)
Flexion malposition	0	1 (IO and graft)

IO = Intertrochanteric osteotomy.

Reoperations in Cases of Femoral Shaft Fractures at the Lower End of the Plate

	CHP arthrodesis (n = 108)	Other techniques (n = 45)
Fatigue fracture without accompanying trauma	0	0
Resulting from accident with or without slight trauma	6	2

All 6 cases healed in the correct position and without complications following osteotomy and compression plate fixation.

With two exceptions, these fractures occurred in the first post-operative months. Treatment of these fractures with a specially long CHP leads to rapid union since the bone turnover rate is high in the first post-operative year and the tendency to heal is therefore marked. Healing was delayed in one of the two fractures which occurred in the second post-operative year. In each case post-operative management of the plate fixation was possible without application of a cast despite the considerable leverage exerted by the leg, and the patient was able to get up after 4 weeks.

Plate fractures: Fracture occurred in 5 of the 107 CHP, 4 as a result of instability of the arthrodesis and 1 following fracture of the femoral neck during the operation.

The cases of instability were: the elderly woman with the infected arthrodesis; the master gardener whose arthrodesis was converted into a total prosthesis; an elderly man who was satisfied with the instability and subsequently died of carcinoma of the stomach, and a woman whose arthrodesis was reo perated and subsequently went on to definitive union.

Fissuring of the femoral neck occurred in a very elderly businessman aged 71 years in whom a CHP arthrodesis was carried out following varusization osteotomy for osteoarthritis. The hip arthrodesis united rapidly since the leverage of the leg was neutralized by the fissuring of the femoral neck. A hip spica was very necessary in this case but was refused by the patient. The inadequate bony support at the level of the femoral neck allowed the leg to exert considerable leverage on the plate and a fatigue fracture of the overloaded plate occurred. The same me-

General Complications

	CHP arthrodesis with PO	Other arthrodeses
	112	45
Post-operative deaths	4	0
Severe pulmonary embolus with good outcome	1	1
Thrombophlebitis	1	2
Carotid artery thrombosis with haemiplegia	1	0
Decubitus	0	3
Extensive evacuation of a haematoma with secondary suturing	2	0
Febrile streptococcal scar infection at 4 or 6 months	2	0
Infection with osteomyelitis	1	0
Femoral nerve paresis (all with full recovery)	6	1
Lateral peroneal nerve paresis with severe residual symptoms	1	1
Lateral peroneal nerve paresis caused by bandage or leg support with recovery	1	1
Paraesthesis originating from lateral cutaneous nerve	3	0

chanism led to fracture in two further CHP despite bony apposition. It took a fourth CHP in combination with correction of an adduction deformity and a hip spica to bring about union.

The CHP arthrodesis combined with PO can be used in a wide range of indications, cast-free post-operative management is possible in 90 % of the cases and the average duration of hospitalization is 44 days. The primary rate of union is similar to that of the best of the other methods available which involve cast fixation and prolonged hospitalization.

In the presence of a simultaneous ipsilateral femoral fracture the CHP will undergo fatigue fracture if no hip spica is applied.

The CHP arthrodesis combined with PO allows individual positioning of the leg. It does not lead to abduction deformity. The mean functional leg length is 0.7 cm less than the true leg length. There is on average, therefore, slight adduction which MERLE D'AUBIGNÉ *et al.* [1964] describes as desirable.

No pain of note is produced in the symphysis and sacroiliac joint by the distortion which results from the PO.

The 4 post-operative deaths following CHP arthrodesis with pelvic osteotomy:

Farmer aged 66 years. Death on 14th post-operative day. Embolus lodged in main pulmonary artery.

Farmer aged 53 years. Death during 6th post-operative week following recurrent pulmonary embolus.

Farmer aged 69 years. Died on 5th post-operative day from cerebral haemorrhage and pulmonary oedema.

Agricultural worker aged 64 years. Cardiac arrest on 6th post-operative day. Patient suffered from bronchiectasis, afebrile bronchopneumonia, myocarditis and acute tumour of the spleen.

The 3.57 % mortality accompanying CHP arthrodesis is not only explained by the severity of the operation. We operated on patients whose poor general condition contraindicated several months of cast fixation.

The infection rate in CHP arthrodesis combined with PO is under 1 %, and is 0.6 % in the total series of 157 arthrodeses. These operations were carried out in the sole operating room which was also used for general surgery.

Transient pareses of the femoral nerve can probably be explained by the pressure exerted by the Hohman retractor during PO and are significantly more frequent following CHP arthrodesis. All cases had recovered after 3 months.

	Back pain			
	before and after opera-tion none, %	post-operative unchanged %	post-operative improve-ment, %	post-opera-tive occur-rence or worsening, %
PADOVANI and JOLY [1951]	60	14	11	15
MERLE D'AUBIGNÉ *et al.* [1964]	47	17	8	28
HÖRDEGEN and TÖNNIS [1970]	46	8	4	42
SCHNEIDER [1972]	57	13	13	17

Back Pain

The picture seen is similar to that accompanying other types of arthrodesis. Only limited comparison of the figures in the following table is possible since the time of observation is variable.

Pelvic tilt should be counteracted by correct positioning of the leg and, if necessary, by shoe blocking in order to prevent post-operative back pain. Worsening of a pre-existing hyperlordosis by positioning the stiffened hip in flexion should be avoided. Severe vertebral insufficiency is a clear contraindication for hip arthrodesis.

Back pain is more marked in large and excessively heavy patients.

The Influence of Hip Arthrodesis on the Opposite Joints

The question of reduction of load on the opposite leg is usually not dealt with in the literature. Accurate positioning of the leg and correct leg length are prerequisites. DEMINGNIEUX *et al.* [1968] assumes that a HA inevitably leads to increased loading of the opposite hip. We cannot agree with this assumption and are supported here by the results of 13 inter-trochanteric osteotomies performed on the opposite hip in cases of bilateral osteoarthritis. The results were as follows: 11 were still functioning after 4–10 years (mean 7.2 years); one was converted into a total prosthesis after 4 years (the indication for osteotomy in this patient was anyway poor: the arthrodesis had itself replaced a 4-year-old osteotomy), and one osteotomy in a young female patient was reosteotomied 7 years after the first osteotomy (HA had been performed 9 years previously).

The results in these intertrochanteric osteotomies suggest that overloading of the opposite hip by an arthrodesis does not occur. The 5-year results were good in 11 out of 13 osteotomies, which is better than average.

Up to 1964, MERLE D'AUBIGNÉ *et al.* had observed 31 cases in which worsening had occured out of a total of 59 cases in which the opposite hip was diseased. They consider this normal for this series, the majority of which were cases of idiopathic osteoarthritis of the hip and states that he has 'never regretted' the arthrodesis of the opposite side.

BOUILLET and DELCHEF [1968] described ipsilateral osteoarthritis of the knee joint following arthrodesis of the hip. We always checked knee function but find nothing in our data to confirm this observation. Axial deformity at the knee joint, abduction deformity of the hip, prolonged cast fixation and internal rotation deformity are mentioned as being the major causes.

In 1969, RUMIANTSEVA expressed the opinion that arthrodesis of the more severely affected side protected the opposite side in cases of bilateral osteoarthritis of the hip.

DEI POLI and FIANDACA [1970] investigated walking, climbing stairs and sitting following arthrodesis of a hip joint. They particularly draw attention to the overloading of the opposite hip joint which occurs during walking if the hips are arthrodesed in excessive extension and to the overloading of the vertebral column and ipsilateral knee joint if excessive flexion is present. Sitting and stair climbing are rendered more difficult by extension and easier by flexion.

Pain Caused by Areas of High Bone Turnover
around the Obturator Foramen

GSCHWEND [1967] described 3 cases in which areas of high bony turnover in the ischiopubic ramus caused pain. They healed following immobilization. It is possible that there is less stress in this area following CHP arthrodesis combined with PO. Again, MERLE D'AUBIGNÉ *et al.* [1964] reported fissuring of the bone in this region following trivial trauma. The fissures all healed. We have never observed this condition.

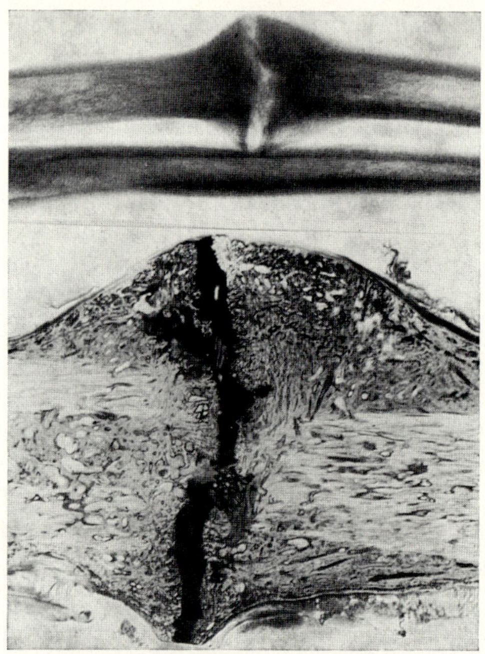

Fig. 16. 40-week-old radial pseudarthrosis produced experimentally in the dog. Fibrous cartilage between the bone ends.

Observations on the Pathophysiology of Hip Arthrodesis

It is clear from study of the various hip arthrodesis techniques that so-called preparation of the joint surfaces, in which cancellous bone is exposed, does not increase the chances of bony union. On the contrary, the increased disturbance of the blood supply to the head of the femur which results from the Charnley method leads to a relatively high non-union rate despite the use of lag screws and cast. A thin superior head segment was resected in approximately half the cases in which a CHP arthrodesis was performed in combination with PO. It was frequently removed and frequently left for congruence reasons. The chances of bony

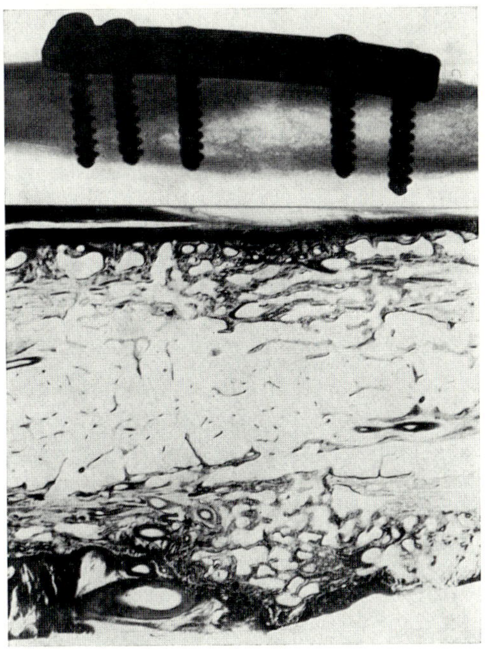

Fig. 17. Similar case. Stabilization for 24 weeks results in bony union, breakdown of the periosteal callus and restoration of the medullary cavity. A large proportion of the strain passes through the excessively large plate and this causes functional adaptation of the cortex which converts to cancellous bone [MÜLLER *et al.,* 1968].

union do not seem to be affected by this latter procedure. The degree of stability is decisive. In an arthrodesis the same phenomenon occurs as that seen in a pseudarthrosis, an experimental example of which is shown in figures 16 and 17. It has long been known from clinical experience that excision of a pseudarthrosis is not necessary. Stabilization by compression arthrodesis, with retention of an adequate blood supply, leads to rapid bony union [MÜLLER and ALLGÖWER 1958]. Immobilization of the osteoarthritic joint cartilage by the stable CHP compression fixation causes the cartilage to become brittle and calcified. Formation of haversian systems occurs and the result is bony union. *It is important to emphasize at this point that the laws of healing of pseudarthrosis also apply to arthrodesis.*

Summary

The problem of hip arthrodesis is discussed. The area and viability of the uniting bony surfaces and the stability of fixation are decisive. Cobra head plate arthrodesis in combination with pelvic osteotomy brings about tension band fixation and produces compression over the whole surface of contact. The result is a large area of stabilizing interfragmentary friction and the uniting bony surfaces are free of implant material. The medialization of the pelvis and femur which is brought about by pelvic osteotomy allows the cobra head plate to be adapted to the prevailing anatomy. The medialization enlarges the area of bony contact and counteracts dislocating forces.

112 cobra head plate arthrodeses performed by us in combination with pelvic osteotomy are compared with 45 cases of hip arthrodesis in which other techniques were used.

The use of the cobra head plate arthrodesis technique allowed the indication for hip arthrodesis to be extended. Infected osteoarthropathies with fistulae and osteolysis were operated, together with elderly patients in whom cast fixation was out of question. 90 % of the patients got out of bed and commenced partial weight bearing after 3 weeks without any cast fixation whatsoever. Despite these factors, which render comparison with other methods difficult, a primary bone union rate of 87 % was obtained. The mean duration of hospital stay was 44 days.

Our results with cobra head plate arthrodesis and pelvic osteotomy confirm our finding in surgery of the extremities that stable internal fixation is the treatment of choice in infected cases as long as the bone is still viable. The head is not dislocated during cobra head plate arthrodesis with pelvic osteotomy and exposure of the cancellous bone of the joint is not carried out. This assures minimum damage of the blood supply of the head. The pathophysiology of bony union in a stably fixed osteoarthritic joint is analogous to that of the healing of a hypervascular pseudarthrosis produced simply by stabilization without resection of the intervening tissue. This reaction of a pseudarthrosis to compression has been adequately demonstrated, both in animal experiments and in clinical practice.

References

Ahlbäck, S.-O. and Lindahl, O.: Hip arthrodesis. The connection between function and position. Acta orthop. scand. *37:* 77–87 (1966).

Albee, F. H.: Arthritis deformans of hip; report of a new operation. J. amer. med. Ass. *50:* 1553–1554 (1908).

Albert, E.: Einige Fälle von künstlicher Ankylosenbildung an paralytischen Gliedmassen. Wien. med. Presse *23:* 725–728 (1882).

Alvik, I.: Arthrodesis of the hip. A method allowing weightbearing and walking postoperatively. Acta orthop. scand. *32:* 451–456 (1962).

Artst, V. A.: Surgical fixation of the hip joint (Russian). Orthop. Travm. Protez. *31:* 51–53 (1970).

AXER, A.: Compression arthrodesis of the hip joint. J. Bone Jt Surg. *43A:* 492–504 (1961).

BAUMANN, F. und BEHR, O.: Elektromyographische Untersuchungen der Hüftmuskulatur nach Arthrodese. Arch. orthop. Unfall-Chir. *66:* 1–17 (1969).

BLAIMONT, P.: Libération d'une arthrodèse ancienne de la hanche par arthroplastie, pour traitement d'une arthrose du genou. Acta orthop. belg. *34:* 983–990 (1968).

BLIETZ, R. und BORGMANN, F.: Die Druckosteosynthese der Hüfte bei Verlust des coxalen Femurendes. Arch. orthop. Unfall-Chir. *62:* 23–28 (1967).

BOUILLET, R. et DELCHEF, J.: L'arthrose du genou, conséquence éloignée de l'ankylose de la hanche. Acta orthop. belg. *34:* 947–968 (1968).

BRITTAIN, H. A.: Ischio-femoral arthrodesis. J. Bone Jt Surg. *30B:* 642–650 (1948).

BUREAU, R.: A propos d'une technique d'arthrodèse de la hanche. Rev. Chir. orthop. *52:* 569–570 (1966).

CASS, C. A. and DWYER, A. F.: A drilling jig for arthrodesis of the hip. J. Bone Jt Surg. *51B:* 135–139 (1969).

CENNI, F.: L'artrodesi nella cura dell'anca paralitica. Chir. Organi. Mov. *55:* 96–111 (1966).

CHAN, K. P. and SHIN, J. S.: Brittain ischiofemoral arthrodesis for tuberculosis of the hip. J. Bone Jt Surg. *50A:* 1341–1352 (1968).

CHAPCHAL, G.: Die Arthrodese des Hüftgelenkes. Chir. Praxis *3:* 65–74 (1959).

CHARNLEY, J.: Treatment of mono-articular arthritis of the hip by the central dislocation operation. J. Bone Jt Surg. *38B:* 592–593 (1956).

CHITRANJAN, S. R.; JORDAN, L. R., and WILSON, P. D.: A technique of muscle-pedicle bone graft in hip arthrodesis. J. Bone Jt Surg. *53A:* 925–934 (1971).

DECOULX, P.; DECOULX, J. et DELBREIL, P.: Une technique d'arthrodèse de la hanche. Acta orthop. belg. *31:* 770–779 (1965).

DEMIANOW, V. M.: Internal fixator for arthrodesis of the hip joint (Russian). Ortop. Travm. Protez. *31:* 70–72 (1970).

DEMIGNEUX, F.; RAINAUT, J.-J. et CÉDART, C.: Etude de la hanche opposée aux arthrodèses. Rev. chir. orthop. *54:* 649–656 (1968).

DICKSON, J. A. and HARTMANN, J. T.: Follow-up notes on articles previously published in the journal. J. Bone Jt Surg. *47A:* 1070–1072 (1965).

DREYER, J. und PINGEL, P.: Unsere Erfahrungen bei der Hüftarthrodese mit Beckenosteotomie und Kreuzplatte. Arch. orthop. Unfall-Chir. *66:* 310–323 (1969).

FARKAS, A.: A new operative treatment of tuberculosis coxitis in children; cited in LIPSCOMB and McCASLIN (1961).

FICHTNER, H. J.: Die Stellungskontrolle bei der Hüftgelenkarthrodese mit Hilfe eines neuen Zweiebenen-Winkelmessers. Z. Orthop. *105:* 263–265 (1969).

GARDINER, T. B.: Nail and graft arthrodesis of the hip. J. Bone Jt Surg. *44B:* 588–594 (1962).

GERTSCH, R.: Die Arthrodese des Hüftgelenks mit Kreuzplatte und Beckenosteotomie. Helv. chir. Acta *33:* 216–221 (1966).

GOESSENS, H.; PINGEL, P. et DREYER, J.: L'arthrodèse de hanche par plaque en croix (cobra head plate arthrodesis). Acta orthop. belg. *36:* 350–361 (1970).

GÖRDES, W.: Erfahrungen mit der Technik der Hüftarthrodese nach Axer-Viernstein. Arch. orthop. Unfall-Chir. *67:* 355–366 (1970).

GÖRDES, W.; VIERNSTEIN, K. und KLEMENT, I.: Erfahrungen mit der Hüftarthrodese nach der AO-Technik. Arch. orthop. Unfall-Chir. *70:* 304–319 (1971).

GSCHWEND, N.: Eine wenig bekannte Komplikation der Hüftarthrodese oder die van Necksche Krankheit des Erwachsenen. Arch. orthop. Unfall-Chir. *62:* 263–267 (1967).

HANSLIK, L. und FRIEDEBOLD, G.: Die Indikationsstellung zur Hüftarthrodese nach Entwicklung stabiler Alloarthroplastiken. Arch. orthop. Unfall-Chir. *68:* 325–342 (1970).

HASS, J.: Extraartikuläre Ankylosierung der Hüfte. Zbl. Chir. *1922:* 1466–1467.

HENSSGE, J.: Geschlossene Hüftgelenksarthrodese mit Knochendübel und verbundener Doppelschraube. Arch. orthop. Unfall-Chir. *61:* 26–29 (1967).

HÖRDEGEN, K. M. und TÖNNIS, D.: Der Einfluss der Hüftgelenks-Arthrodese auf die Wirbelsäule. Arch. orthop. Unfall-Chir. *69:* 97–113 (1970).

KALÉN, R.: Internal fixation in hip joint arthrodesis. Experimental studies in autopsy specimens. Acta orthop. scand. *112:* suppl. (1968).

LAM, S. J. S.: Arthrodesis of the hip. With special reference to early mobilisation without external splintage. J. Bone Jt Surg. *50B:* 14–23 (1968).

LANGE, M.: Arthrodesis of the hip. Review of a series of more than five hundred cases. J. int. Coll. Surg. *29:* 638–643 (1958).

LANGENSKIÖLD, A. and LAURENT, L. E.: Compression arthrodesis of the hip joint by the method of Axer. Acta orthop. scand. *38:* 359–367 (1967).

LINDAHL, O.: Determination of hip adduction, especially in arthrodesis. Acta orthop. scand. *36:* 280–293 (1965).

LIPSCOMB, P. R. and McCASLIN, F. E.: Arthrodesis of the hip. Review of 371 cases. J. Bone Jt Surg. *43A:* 923–938 (1961).

MERLE d'AUBIGNÉ, R. J.; RAMADIER, O.; POSTEL, M.; MAZAS, F. et VAILLANT, J.-M.: L'arthrodèse de la hanche. Rev. Chir. orthop. *50:* 789–812 (1964).

MITTELMEIER, H.: Druckarthrodese der Hüfte. 15. Tagung der Med.-wissenschaftl. Ges. für Orthopädie in der DDR (1966).

MONTMOLLIN, B. DE: Arthrodèse de la hanche. Technique et résultat. Helv. chir. acta *35:* 130–132 (1968).

MORRIS, J. B.: Charnley compression arthrodesis of the hip. J. Bone Jt Surg. *48B:* 260–279 (1966).

MÜLLER, B. S.: Kompressionsarthrodese des Hüftgelenkes. Beitr. Orthop. *15:* 149–151 (1968).

MÜLLER, J.; SCHENK, R. und WILLENEGGER, H. W.: Experimentelle Untersuchungen über die Entstehung reaktiver Pseudoarthrosen am Hunderadius. Helv. chir. Acta *35:* 301–308 (1968).

MÜLLER, M. E.: Die hüftnahen Femurosteotomien; 2. Aufl. (Thieme, Stuttgart 1971).

MÜLLER, M. E.: Personal communication (1961).

MÜLLER, M. E.: Personal communication (1964).

MÜLLER, M. E. und ALLGÖWER, M.: Zur Behandlung der Pseudarthrosen. Helv. chir. Acta *25:* 356–364 (1958).

ONJI, Y.; KURATA, Y., and KIDO, H.: A new method of hip fusion using an intramedullary nail. J. Bone Jt Surg. *47B:* 690–693 (1965).

PADOVANI, P. et JOLY, J.-P.: Résultats éloignés de 308 arthrodèses de hanche. Rev. Chir. orthop. *47:* 83–89 (1951).

POLI, N. DEI e FIANDACA, A.: Fisiopatologia delle articolazioni di compenso nell'artrodesi d'anca. Minerva ortop. *21:* 81–88 (1970).

RADULESCU, A. D.: Nouveau procédé de verrouillage de la hanche arthrosique douloureuse. Rev. Chir. orthop. *49:* 623–624 (1963).

RATOMSKI, R.; JESKE, W.; ADAMCZEWSKI, J, und HABRYCH, A.: Die operative Hüftarthrodese nach Müller. Beitr. Orthop. *17:* 113–116 (1970).

RUMIANTSEVA, A. A.: Compression arthrodesis in bilateral coxarthrosis (Russian with Enlish summary). Ortop. Travm. Protez. *30:* 37–40 (1969).

SCHNEIDER, R.: Technik der Hüftarthrodese mit Beckenosteotomie und Kreuzplatte. Arch. klin. Chir. *316:* 233 (1966).

SCHOTTEN, P.: Hüftgelenksarthrodese mit einer Federringschraube in Kombination mit intertrochantärer Osteotomie und Hüftgelenksplombierung. Arch. orthop. Unfall-Chir. *60:* 274–280 (1966).

SHIKITA, T.; AZUMA, T., and KAKIMOTO, T.: Compression fixation of the femoral head by transarticular nailing (Japanese with English summary). Iryo, Tokyo *24:* 873–882 (1970).

SOMERVILLE, E. W.: Two-nail fixation of the hip. J. Bone Jt Surg. *51B:* 648–653 (1969).

STEWART, M. J. and COKER, T. P.: Arthrodesis of the hip. A review of 109 patients. Clin. Orthop. *62:* 136–150 (1969).

TEINTURIER, P.: Arthrodèse de la hanche. Lambeau pédiculé trochantérien avec vissage ischio-fémoral. Rev. Chir. orthop. *52:* 645–649 (1966).

THOMPSON, F. R.: Combined hip fusion and subtrochanteric osteotomy allowing early ambulation; cited in LIPSCOMB and MCCASLIN (1961).

VESELY, D. G.: Ischiofemoral arthrodesis. An end-result study of fourty-four cases. J. Bone Jt Surg. *43A:* 363–378 (1961).

VIERNSTEIN, K. und WEIGERT, M.: Fortschritte in der Technik der Arthrodese. Münch. med. Wschr. *110:* 829–837 (1968).

WATSON-JONES, R. and ROBINSON, W. C.: Arthrodesis of the osteoarthritic hip joint. J. Bone Jt Surg. *38B:* 353–377 (1956).

WILKINSON, M. C.: Intertrochanteric osteotomy for the treatment of tuberculosis of the hip; cited in LIPSCOMB and MCCASLIN (1961).

Author's address: Dr. med. ROBERT SCHNEIDER, Chirurg FMH, Alpenstrasse 15, *CH-2500 Biel* (Schweiz)

Reconstr. Surg. Traumat., vol. 14, pp. 38–64 (Karger, Basel 1974)

Fractures of the Shaft of the Humerus
An Analysis of 100 Consecutive Cases

W. HOSNER

Accident Hospital of the General Injuries Insurance Company
(Medical Director: A. TITZE), Graz

Contents

Even nowadays fracture management does not always give satisfactory results. It is hoped that by this statistical study the causes of failures might be better understood. In this paper all data and medical records of a consecutive series of 100 cases of fractures of the humeral shaft, treated in this hospital during the years 1956–1960, are analysed. Seven cases appertaining to this period in which the fractures of the humeral shaft were associated with other severe injuries and of whom 4 patients died soon after admission and the remaining 3 patients had a long recumbency, were not included into this study. Infratubercular fractures and epidiacondylar fractures of the humerus were also excluded.

Of our 100 cases 88 had closed fractures and 12 had open fractures. 55 cases were classified as accidents of work.

Noteworthy are the large numbers of falls on level ground, just as the numbers of avulsion injuries; the latter can easily be avoided by proper safeguard equipment. Taking into account the severity of avulsion injuries – as extensive skin damage and soft tissue damage – such safety fittings are surely justified.

Of our 100 cases 58 had fractures of the left arm and 42 of the right arm. 69 were males and 31 females.

The relatively large number of injured children and juveniles is remarkable, the more so as the cases from the Graz Children's Hospital have not been taken into account. It seems that children are more subject to accidents because of their sporting activity. The frequency in elderly people may be related to other causes such as osteoporosis and arthrosis.

Treatment

Treatment was mainly conservative as advocated by Böhler. After appropriate physical examination of the patient, whereby special attention should be paid to nerve injuries, X-ray photographs are taken in two planes. Then gentle manipulated reduction is performed under local anaesthesia with the patient sitting and a plaster cast is applied to maintain

Table I. Mechanism of injury

	Number of cases
Fall on level ground	39
Traffic accidents	25
Sudden fall from a height	15
Injuries by direct force	12
Avulsion injuries	9
(caused by transmission belts,	
gear wheels and moving rollers)	
	100

Table II. Age distribution (average age 38 years)

Age, years	Number of cases
5–10	6
10–20	25
20–30	15
30–40	11
40–50	11
50–60	9
60–70	12
70–80	9
80–90	2
	100

reduction. An angulation of 20° is tolarated at primary reduction, for 3 weeks later the plaster cast has to be changed anyway. When callus formation has set in and soft tissue swelling has subsided final reduction (alignment) can be performed more easily. Elongation must be avoided, whereas slight shortening is desirable. The kind of immobilisation depends on the site of fracture and partly also on the age group (child or adult). Fractures in the proximal third are generally immobilised by a Desault plaster cast or a U-shaped plaster splint. In fractures of the distal third a palm-to-shoulder plaster cast is applied. This plaster has to be split (bivalved) immediately after setting. Fractures in the middle third are generally immobilised by a U-shaped plaster splint. However, children with such fractures are immobilised by a Desault plaster cast (fig. 1–3). All plaster casts are non-padded. X-ray photographs are taken immedi-

Table III. Characteristics of fractures

Characteristic	Number of cases
Type or pattern of fracture	
Spiral fractures and long oblique fractures	43
Transversal fractures and short oblique fractures	17
Bending fractures (with intermediate butterfly fragment) and compound fractures	40
	100
Site or level of fracture	
Proximal third	20
Middle third	60
Distal third	20
	100
Dislocation and shortening	
Gross dislocation (more than shaft diameter) and considerable shortening	29
Slight dislocation and slight shortening	71
	100

ately after application of plaster. Further roentgenographs are taken a week later and then in 2-week intervals until removal of plaster cast. A final X-ray picture is taken at the end of treatment. The time of immobilisation varies according to the age group and the type of fracture. As a rule, a period of 5–6 weeks is sufficient for healing in children, whereas in adults an immobilisation of 8 weeks is generally required. Transverse fractures with little contact need 1–2 weeks more to consolidate. After removing the plaster cast the consolidation of fracture has to be verified. Here the clinical findings are usually more important than X-ray pictures. If the fracture has not consolidated, another plaster cast is applied for an additional period of 2–4 weeks. All patients are instructed to exercise all non-immobilised joints.

Patients with open fractures or radial nerve lesions are always hospitalised. The same applies to patients who live far outside town. After removal of the plaster cast active exercises are instituted as well as hydrotherapy. Two weeks later physical therapy and passive exercises are begun. Open fractures are treated in the same way as closed fractures after wound excision and suturing have been carried out. Here the plaster cast has not only to be split (bivalved) but also windowed over the wound. If

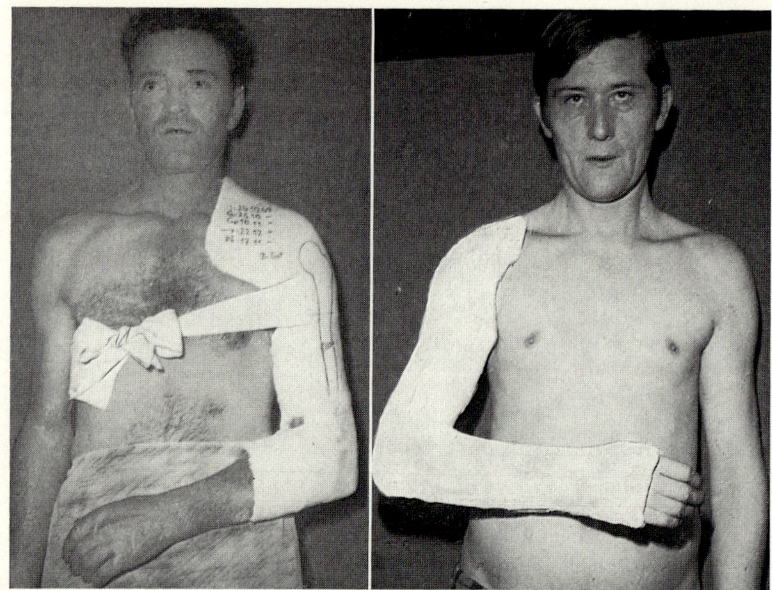

1, 2

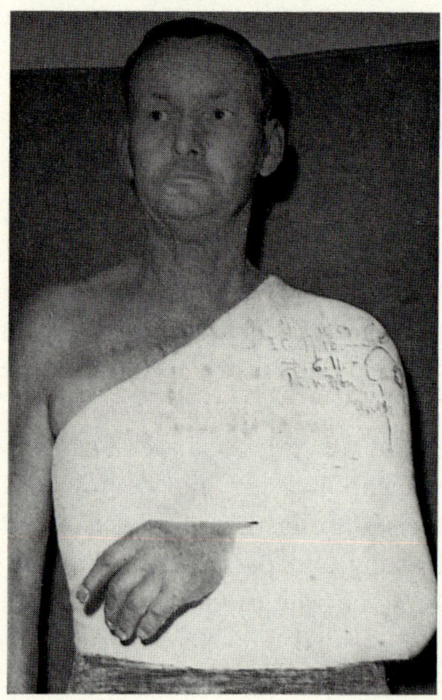

3

Fig. 1. U-shaped plaster splint.
Fig. 2. Palm-to-shoulder cast.
Fig. 3. Desault's plaster cast.

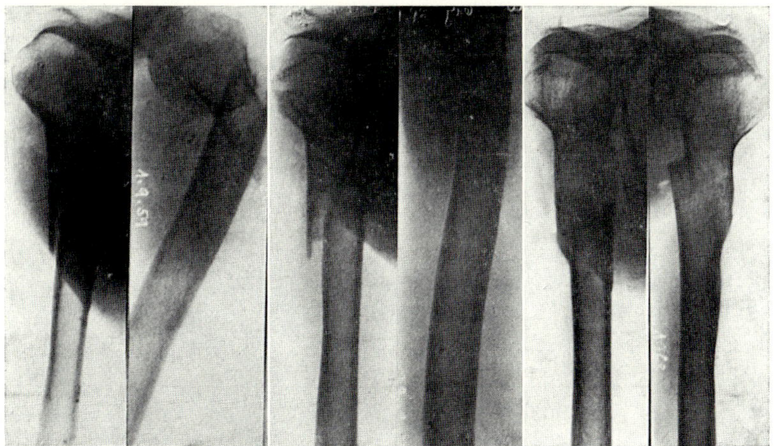

Fig. 4. Case No. 60. Farmer, aged 61. Fracture in the proximal third of the humerus. Immobilisation in Desault's plaster cast for 4 weeks. Two months after removal of plaster limitation of shoulder 130°. Nine years later only 30°.

radial nerve injury is present in an open fracture, a primary exploration of the nerve is carried out and if necessary a nerve suture is performed (at present we would usually carry out an ostesynthesis at the same time). In closed fractures with radial nerve damage the exploration of he nerve is usually delayed for 3 months, because we know by experience that many nerve lesions recover spontaneously.

Table IV shows that solid union occurred within 8 weeks in 65 % and within 10 weeks in 81 % of all patients. In 89 % of our patients the fractures had been consolidated 12 weeks after injury. We had only 1 case of re-fracture (No. 32), of which details will be given later. There were 2 cases of non-union (No. 7 and 84) which will also be discussed later. It may be said in general that an average of 61 days was found to be an adequate period of immobilisation.

Our 100 patients together wore plaster casts for a total time of 6,101 days; namely U-shaped splints for 3,682 days (approx. 60 %), palm-to-shoulder casts for 1,783 days (approx. 30 %) and Desault's casts for 636 days (approx. 10 %).

There was no apparent correlation between the different age groups and the required time of immobilisation. In children only the fractures healed 1–3 weeks earlier than in adults.

The average time of hospital stay of the above 65 patients was 18 days, that is 12 days related to 100 cases. 35 patients were not admitted and were treated as out-patients.

Table IV. Time of immobilisation in plaster cast

Time in weeks	Number of cases (or %)
4– 6	22
6– 8	43
8–10	16
10–12	8
More than 12	11
	100

64 of our patients were workmen or employees or independent contractors or farmers. They returned to work at an average of 105 days and their after-treatment was discontinued at an average of 107 days after injury. 36 patients had no occupation (housewives, pupils, pensioners, etc.). Their average time of treatment lasted 113 days. This disproves the general opinion that the majority of injured workers tried to delay return to work. It is true, however, that more than 40 % of the patients had not resumed work 14 weeks after injury.

One patient, a white collar worker resumed work on the very day of injury, after reduction had been carried out and a plaster cast had been applied.

Surgical Treatment

Two of the 12 patients with open fractures had only small wounds of 1–2 cm in length (i. e. skin perforations caused by a sharp fracture fragment). These two cases were treated in the usual conservative way after the wounds had been cleaned and covered with a sterile ointment pad. In eight other cases the wounds were 3–10 cm long. They were excised and sutured. There was one infection with drainage and following sequester formation. Six months after injury a sequestrotomy was carried out on this patient (case No. 22) and after that drainage subsided.

In two other cases skin grafting was required owing to skin defects 6 × 6 cm in extent. Partial necrosis of these skin grafts necessitated secondary skin grafting 6–9 weeks after injury (case No. 95 and 17).

Two of the open fractures were actually avulsion fractures with extensive skin loss and soft tissue loss. In case No. 77 the necrtic tissue

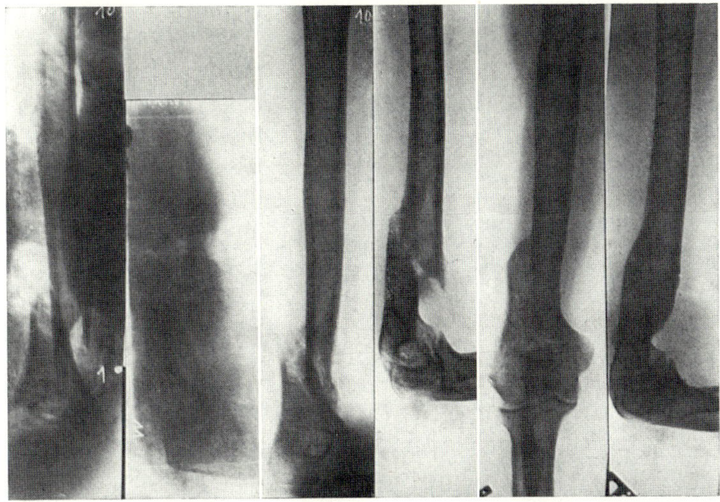

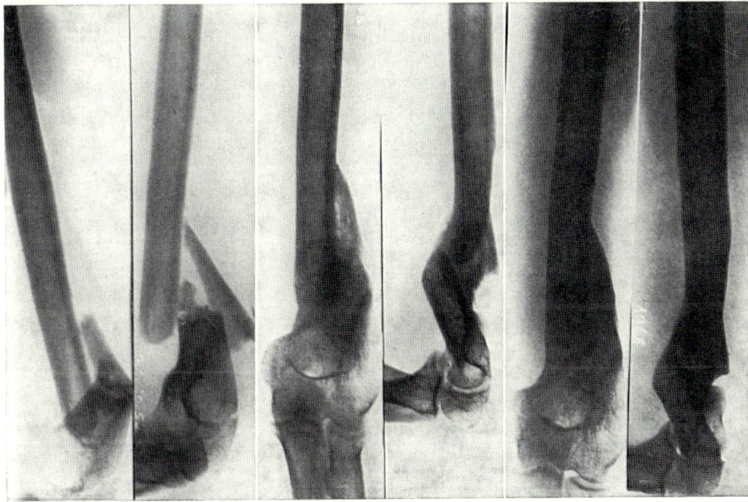

Fig. 5. Case No. 10. House-wife, aged 37. Fracture of the right humerus in the distal third. Immobilisation for 3 weeks in Desault's plaster cast and then for another 5 weeks in U-shaped plaster splint. Eleven weeks after removal of plaster the elbow joint was impaired 70°. Twelve years later 25°.

Fig. 6. Case No. 6. White collar worker, aged 30. Open fracture of the left humerus in the distal third. Wound excision and sutures. Immobilisation by U-shaped plaster splint for 7 weeks. Five weeks after removal of plaster a limitation of elbow motion of 40° and a limitation of pronation and supination in the forearm of one third was noted. Twelve years later same findings.

Table V. Kind of plaster casts applied

Plaster cast	Number of cases
U-shaped splints	57
Palm-to-shoulder casts	22
Desault's casts	7
Two or three of the above casts successively	14
	100

Table VI. Advantages and disadvantages of the three different types of plaster casts used

Plaster cast	Advantage	Disadvantage
U-shaped splint (fig. 1)	small weight and no elongation	immobilisation incomplete
Palm-to-shoulder cast (fig. 2)	good immobilisation for fractures in the distal third	weighty (i. e. traction on the fracture fragments). Insufficient for fractures in the prox. and middle third
Desault's plaster cast (fig. 3)	ideal immobilisation (adjacent joints included). No traction on the fracture fragments as the cast is supported by the shoulder	heavy and oppressing. Risk of temporary shoulder stiffness in elderly people

Table VII. Duration of hospitalisation

Time, weeks	Cases	Percent
Less than one	31	48
1–3	17	26
3–8	12	18
More than eight	5	8
	65	100

Table VIII. Duration of ambulatory treatment (average 97 days)

Time, weeks	Number of cases
Less than 10	35
10–12	14
12–14	24
More than 14	27

Average total time of treatment 109 days (12 plus 97).

Table IX. Return to work after injury

Time, weeks	Cases	Percent
Within ten	15	23
10–12	11	17
12–14	12	19
Later than 14	26	41
	64	100

Table X. Angulation and dislocation of fracture after consolidation

	Number of cases
Angulation	
Less than 10°	65
10–20°	32
More than 20°	3
	100
Dislocation	
Less than shaft diameter	73
More than shaft diameter	27
	100
Shortening	
0–10 mm	71
10–20 mm	20
More than 20 mm	9
	100

in the wound was excised and the severed veins ligated. A relaxion incision was required to close the wound, and the remaining skin defect was covered by skin graft. A Desault plaster cast was applied and the wound healed primarily. Three months after injury homologous bone grafting was carried out and the bone fragments were stabilised by a wire loop, as delayed union had become obvious (at the present time we would use another kind of osteosynthesis). At the same time the radial nerve was explored as a radial palsy had developed. The nerve was found impacted in a bed of callus and scar tissue, but otherwise intact. It recovered nearly completely after it had been mobilised and placed in healthy tissue. Solid union occurred with an angulation of 25°. Shoulder motion and elbow motion was impaired ²/₃ when the patient resumed work 9 months after injury. The final result, however, has been satisfactory.

In the second case of avulsion fracture (No. 95), shock was present at admission; this forbade immediate surgery. Therefore, the wound was initially only rinsed with 1 % Cetavlon solution and covered with sterile dressings. A padded metal splint was applied. Surgical treatment was deferred to the following day, according to the principles discussed by ISELIN. Then the wound was excised and the bone fragments were stabilised by a wire loop, then the severed radial nerve was sutured and a skin graft was carried out. The arm was immobilised by a Desault plaster cast. Here wound healing was delayed by partial skin necrosis and transistory drainage. The nerve recovered only gradually. The final result is unknown.

In another case (No. 1) exploration of the radial nerve was carried out 3 months after injury, because of persisting palsy. The impacted nerve was injected by 0.9 % sodium solution and removed from its bed into healthy tissue. Complete recovery resulted. In a further case (No. 37) homologous bone grafting was carried out because of delayed union.

Early Results

Range of Motion of Shoulder

At the time when treatment was ended 43 patients of our series had no or only a slight limitation of abduction of shoulder (less than 25°).

36 patients had a functional limitation of more than 30°. 21 patients failed to attend before completion of treatment and therefore their range of motion is unknown. 22 of the 36 patients mentioned above with a

considerable limitation of motion of shoulder had their plaster casts removed just a few weeks before.

Two months after removal of plaster (or later) 5 patients had a limitation of motion of more than 90° and 6 patients a limitation of 60–85°. These initial results seem to be very unfavourable. The final results, however, which will be discussed later, do not note a single case of marked limitation of shoulder motion. The average age of our 11 patients with initial considerable limitation of shoulder was 54 years (average in total series 38 years). They had plaster casts applied for an average of 71 days (61 days in total series). None of them had a palm-to-shoulder cast. Four had a Desault cast and 7 a U-shaped splint. From this it might be concluded that a limitation of shoulder is favoured by old age and by plaster casts which immobilise the shoulder (Desault's cast and U-shaped splint, which also impedes shoulder motion owing to a sling to the opposite axilla). There was no relation found between level of fracture and limitation of shoulder.

Range of Motion of Elbow at the End of Treatment

In 71 patients of our series the range of motion is mentioned in the records, when treatment was ended. Two months after removal of plaster or later 6 patients had a limitation of motion between 70 and 100°. Four of them had fractures in the distal third of the humerus and three of them were immobilised in a plaster cast for more than 4 months. Two patients in this group had also a considerable limitation of shoulder. It seems that the age did not influence the limitation of elbow motion in adults, the average of the group of six being 34 years (38 years in the total series).

In general it might be said that by reduction and immobilisation in plaster casts only the angulation had been improved but not, however, lateral dislocation.

Radial Nerve Lesion

Radial nerve lesions were noted in ten of our series of 100 cases. Course and details of these 10 cases are shown in table XI.

In 10 cases with radial nerve lesion (table XI) there remained only 1 case with complete radial nerve palsy (No. 58). Among the 5 cases

Table XI. Radial nerve lesion

Case No.	Age years	Clinical findings after injury		Conservative therapy	Surgical therapy			Findings at the end of treatment		
		fall hand	sensory impairment		interval between injury and treatment	findings at surgical intervention	surgical procedure	interval between injury and follow-up, months	fall hand	sensory impairment
1	13	yes	yes	physical therapy	3 months	nerve inconspicious	injection of nerve with sodium solution 0.9 %	5	no	no
16	18	yes	no	B-vitamins palsy plint	–	–	–	2	no	no
38	38	yes	yes	B-vitamins palsy splint	–	–	–	2	no	slight
71	19	no	no	–	–	–	–	3	no	slight
72	35	no	no	B-vitamins owing to secondary noted sensory impairment	–	–	–	2	no	no

Table XI (continued)

Case No.	Age years	Clinical findings after injury		Conservative therapy	Surgical therapy			Findings at the end of treatment		
		fall hand	sensory impairment		interval between injury and treatment	findings at surgical intervention	surgical procedure	interval between injury and follow-up, months	fall hand	sensory impairment
77	32	yes	yes	B-vitamins palsy splint	3 months	nerve impacted in scar tissue	nerve moved into healthy tissue	9	very slight	very slight
87	10	no	no	B-vitamins owing to secondary noted sensory impairment	–	–	–	3	no	no
95	7	yes	yes	–	1 day	nerve severed	nerve suture	6	partly	slight
22	6	no	slight	–	6 months	nerve impacted in scar tissue	nerve moved into healthy tissue	8	no	slight
58	22	yes	no	–	3 months	nerve severed (deficiency 2 inch)	nerve suture failed; second. substit. tendon transplant.	12	partly	yes

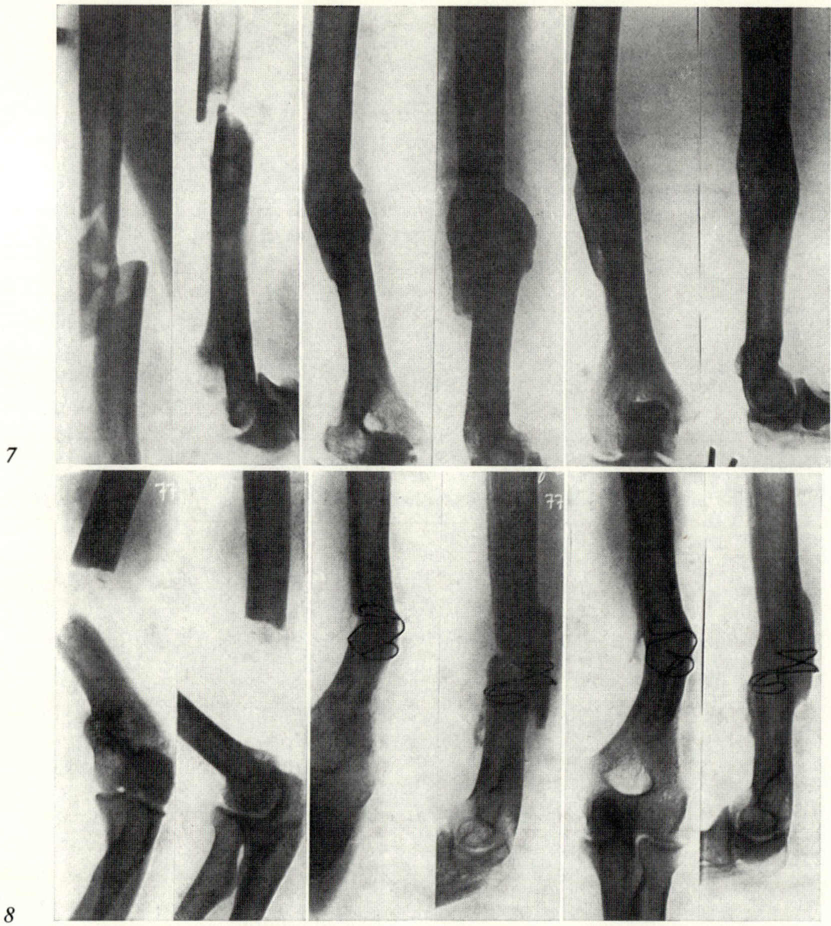

Fig. 7. Case No. 25. Carpenter, aged 44. Spiral fracture of the right humerus in the middle third. Immobilisation by U-shaped plaster splint for 8 weeks. Eleven years later all arm joints were found unimpaired. However, an atrophy of muscles with a deficiency in circumference of 1 in was noted.

Fig. 8. Case No. 77. Foreman, aged 32. Avulsion fracture of the left humerus. Wound excision and suturing plus skin grafting. Immobilisation in Desault's plaster cast. Wound healing uneventful. Three months after injury surgical intervention owing to persisting radial nerve palsy and delayed union. Exploration and mobilisation of the impacted nerve. Fixation of the bone fragments by means of a wire loop and bone grafting. Immobilisation in Desault's plaster for a period of 20 weeks (!). Nine months after injury limitation of shoulder 120° and impairment of elbow joint 100°. Fracture healing with angulation (varus) of 25°. Radial nerve palsy subsided nearly completely. Late results 8 years after injury: limitation of shoulder 15°, limitation of elbow joint 20°. Pronation and supination of the forearm impaired ¼. Final partial disability 25 %.

which initially showed fall hand, motor impairment subsided completely or gradually: twice by conservative treatment (No. 26 and 38, complete recovery); once after exploration of the nerve and injection with 0.9 % sodium solution (No. 1, complete recovery); once after mobilisation of the nerve (No. 77, gradual recovery: fingers gained full extension, wrist extension remained impaired by $1/3$), and once after suturing of the dissected nerve (No. 95). In the latter case at the end of treatment finger extension was impaired by $3/4$, wrist extension by $1/3$.

At the end of treatment 5 patients showed more or less gradual sensory impairment of the radial nerve. It is interesting to note that in 3 of these 5 cases initially no radial nerve lesion was diagnosed. It became evident during the time of immobilisation in plaster or after removal of plaster. There are two explanations possible: either the nerve impairment failed to cause attention at the initial medical examination or it really occurred secondarily by pressure of the haematome or by damage to the nerve on reduction.

As mentioned above we usually delayed nerve exploration in closed fractures with radial nerve damage for 3 months.

Refracture

In our series we had 1 case of refracture (No. 32). A man, aged 19, sustained an open transversal fracture in the distal third of the humerus. Accessory to this he had a rupure of a kidney which was also treated conservatively. The patient wore a palm-to-shoulder cast for 63 days. Four days after removal of plaster he fell down on level ground on his stretched arm and he sustained a refracture of the humerus. Another palm-to-shoulder plaster cast was applied for 43 days. One month after removal of plaster there was no limitation in shoulder motion and only a very slight limitation of elbow motion.

Non-Union

We had two cases of non-union in our series (No. 7 and 84). Already prior to the fracture, however, case No. 7 had pathological findings on the humerus. The patient was a miner, aged 35, who fell from a ladder in the year 1956 and had his humerus fractured. The same man had already

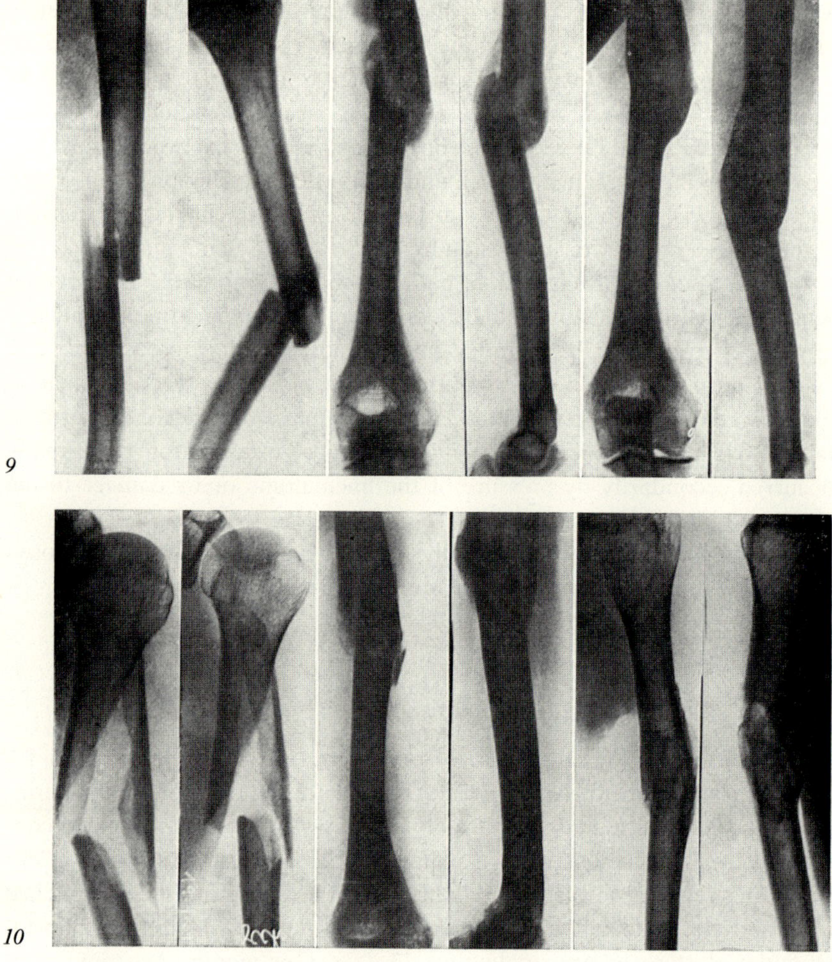

Fig. 9. Case No. 48. Housewife, aged 50. Fracture of the left humerus in the middle third. Immobilisation in U-shaped splint for 9 weeks. Late results 10 years after injury: angulation 20° (varus and antecurvation). No limitation of motion in arm joints.

Fig. 10. Case No. 56. Farmer, aged 55. Fracture of the left humerus. Immobilisation in U-shaped splint for 12 weeks. Fracture healing with angulation of 20°. Late results 9 years after injury: terminal restriction in shoulder and elbow joint. Limitation of pronation and supination in forearm 1/4. Final partial disability 20 %.

sustained a fracture of the humerus in 1944 by a shot, and this sclopetarian fracture had healed with thickening of the bone. After the injury in 1956 the arm was immobilised in a palm-to-shoulder plaster cast for a period of 219 days.

At the end of treatment, 10 months after injury, non-union was evident, though the stability was good and the patient more or less free of complaints. Shoulder movement was only slightly impaired, elbow motion ranged from 140–80° and wrist and finger joints showed no limitation. The final result was good. The non-union healed spontaneously and the function was very good.

The other case (No. 84), a farmer aged 19, fell and sustained a 'butterfly' fracture of the humerus in the middle third while hoisting wood. A U-shaped plaster splint was applied for 12 weeks and the fracture seemed to consolidate with an angulation of 20° varus deformity. Work was resumed 1 month after removal of plaster. A year later the patient complained about pain in his arm. Medical examination revealed non-union, which then was treated surgically by step-like osteotomy and screwing. Uneventful healing.

Delayed Union

In our series we had 7 cases of delayed union (No. 37, 44, 63, 65, 67, 69, and 77). The average time of immobilisation in plaster was 18 weeks and the average time of treatment 25 weeks (in the total series the corresponding figures were 9 and 16 weeks). The meanage of these 7 patients was 46 years (38 years in the total series). Five of these 7 patients had transverse fractures of the humerus in the middle third. Six of them were immobilised by a U-shaped plaster splint and one by a palm-to-shoulder cast. In two of these cases a bone graft was carried out because of delayed union (No. 37 and 77).

Initial Results of Open Fractures of the Humerus

As mentioned before we had in our series 12 cases of open fractures, two of which were avulsion fractures (No. 77 and 95). The average time of treatment in these 12 cases was 155 days (109 days in the whole series) and the average time of hospitalisation was 36 days (12 days in the whole

Table XII. Complications in open fractures (5 out of 12 cases)

Complication	Number of cases
Wound healing impaired by drainage and sequester formation	1
Wound healing complicated by partial necrosis of skingraft and radial nerve palsy	1
Wound healing delayed by partial necrosis of skin graft	1
Delayed union and considerable limitation of shoulder	1
Refracture	1

series). The average time of immobilisation in plaster casts was 68 days (61 days). In 5 cases (40 %) complications were noted as shown in table XII.

Initial Results of Transversal Fractures (and Short Oblique Fractures) of the Humerus

The only case in our series in which refracture occurred was a transversal fracture. Of the 2 cases of non-union one had a transversal fracture. In transversal fractures bone healing was delayed for 1–2 weeks in comparison to other types of fractures. Transversal fractures with dislocation and shortening needed an additional week of immobilisation. None the less, we would like to stress that in transversal fractures good results can also be achieved by conservative treatment.

Other Events and Complications in Convalescence

A patient, aged 55, with atrophic skin sustained a 7-in long plaster cutter injury, which had to be sutured. Several patients had skin lesions caused by pressure of plaster cast which necessitated windowing of casts. Two patients got carbuncles in the armpits while wearing casts.

Summary of Initial Results of Fractures of the Humerus

In our series of 100 cases the initial results were good in 78 (%) but not fully satisfactory in 22 (%) as shown in table XIII.

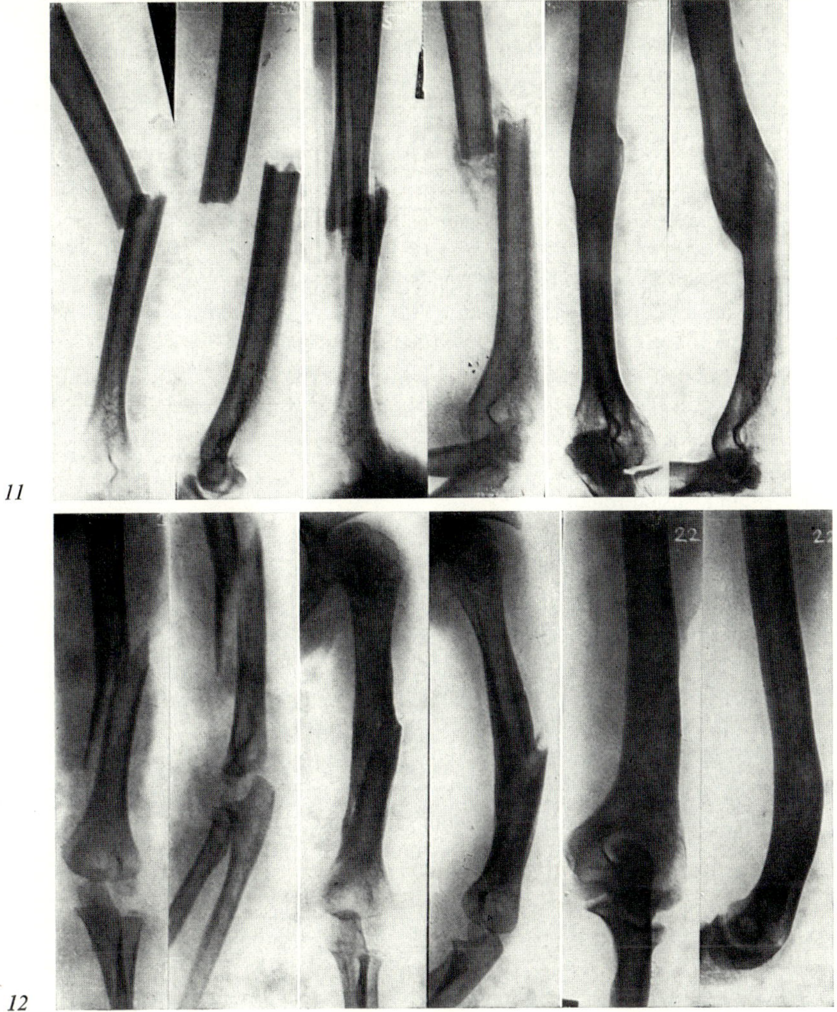

Fig. 11. Case No. 58. Doorkeeper, aged 22. Open fracture of the left humerus with radial nerve palsy. Wound excision and suturing. Palm-to-shoulder cast for 11 weeks. Three months after injury exploration of the radial nerve. Nerve suture failed because of large defect (at present we would carry out a 'cable transplantation' taken from the Nervus suralis). Substitutive tendon graft (Perthes' graft). Fair motor function. Final partial disability 25 %. Radiographs taken 9 years after injury show a progressive angulation. Obviously the period of immobilisation was too short.

Fig. 12. Case No. 22. Child, aged 6. Open spiral fracture of the left humerus. Excision of wound and suturing. Desault's plaster cast. Wound healing complicated by drainage and sequester formation. Removal of sequester and exploration of radial nerve 6 months after injury. Late result 11 years after injury: elbow extension lacking 15°; all other arm joints without limitation. Angulation not grown out.

Table XIII. Poor initial results

Result	Number of cases
Considerable limitation of shoulder Five cases more than 90°, 6 cases 60–90° Favouring circumstances: old age, long immobilisation	11
Limitation of elbow joint (more than 60°) Four of these 6 patients had fractures in the distal third	6
Angulation of more than 25° Two of them had open fractures with impaired wound healing	3
Radial palsy (complete)	1
Gradual motor impairment of the radial nerve Both avulsion fractures	2
Non-union	2
Refracture Transversal fracture	1
Drainage and sequester formation Open fracture	1
Delayed union (immobilisation longer than 18 weeks) Five of these 7 patients had transversal fractures in the middle third	7

These 34 complications occurred in 22 patients.

Apart from the two avulsion fractures, there remain 20 cases (20 %) of un-satisfactory initial results.

Late Results

During the year 1968 we invited all 100 patients with diaphyseal fractures of the humerus to follow-up examination. 20 of them did not reply. Seven were reported as deceased. 20 others were lost to us because of change of address (present address unknown).

53 Patients Attended the Follow-Up Examination

The average age of these 53 patients was 44.5 years, that is 3.5 years above the mean of the total series. This may be explained by the loss of the deceased and the loss of patients who have difficulties in walking; both these groups are comprised of elderly people.

Complaints: Mild Complaints Were Noted in 27 Patients (51 %)

27 patients (about half of our follow-up patients), complained about occasional mild pain in the injured arm, especially during a change of weather. 26 replied to this leading question: 'No, no complaints at all.'

Limitation of Motion of Shoulder: 6 Patients (11 %) 20–50°

Three of the patients hat a limitation of 30–50° (No. 17, 31, 60). Three others had a limitation of 20–25° (No. 18, 41, 86). The extent of limitation is always related to the unimpaired opposite arm. The average age of these 6 patients was 64 years, that is 20 years above the mean of the 53 follow-up patients. It is noteworthy that in this respect early results and late results do not correspond. All our follow-up patients could lift their arms above level.

Limitation of Elbow Joint: 7 Patients (13 %) 25–50°

Three of our follow-up patients had a limitation of 40–50° (No. 6, 7, 31), four others a limitation of 25–30° (No. 10, 37, 83). The majority of them had fractures in the distal third of the humerus. Here early results and late results showed a striking conformity. All patients with considerable limitation of the elbow 2 months after removal of plaster had also a marked limitation of motion in this joint 8–12 years later.

Limitation of Pronation and Supination in the Forearm: 7 Patients (13 %) Showed Impairment of $^{1}/_{4}$–$^{1}/_{2}$

One patient (No. 11) had an impairment of 50 % (approx. 40°). His fracture had healed with an internal rotation of 40°. In two other cases (No. 17 and 22) pronation and supination was impaired one third and in four others (No. 6, 7, 31, 77) one fourth. Three of these 7 patients had fractures in the distal third which had healed with an angulation of 20 to 25° and a dislocation of more than width of shaft.

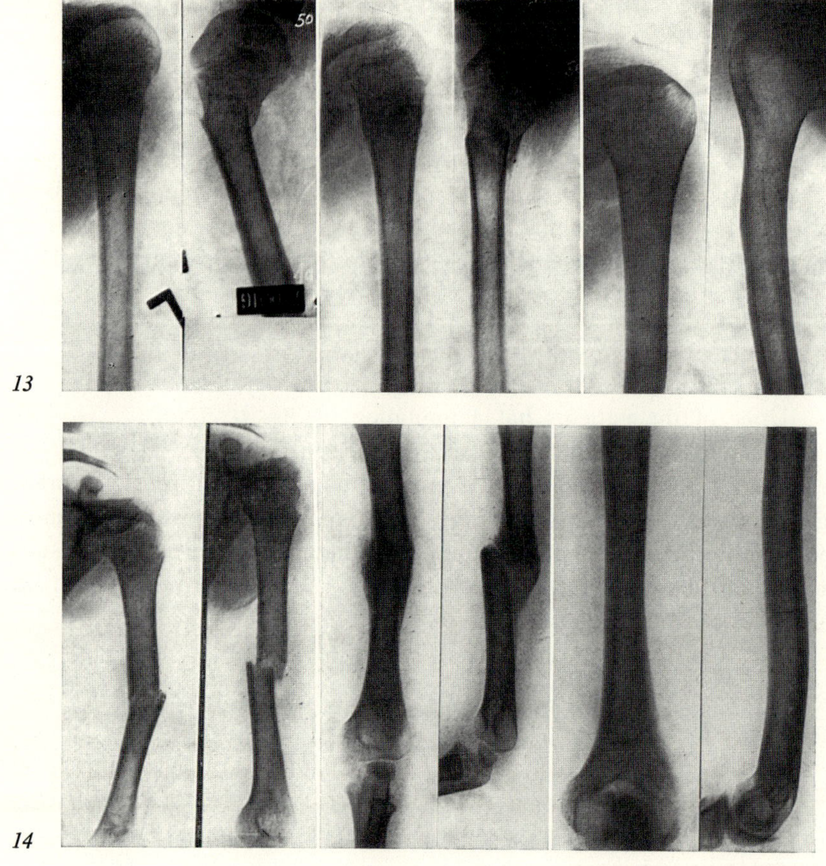

Fig. 13. Case No. 50. Pupil, aged 13. Fracture of the left humeral shaft in the upper third. Immobilisation in Desault's plaster cast for 4 weeks. Ten years after injury angulation 10°. The bending, which was originally subcapital, has shifted by bone growth to the middle third.

Fig. 14. Case No. 14. Child, aged 5. Transversal fracture of the left humerus in the middle third. Palm-to-shoulder cast for 5 weeks. Eleven years after injury dislocation has grown out completely.

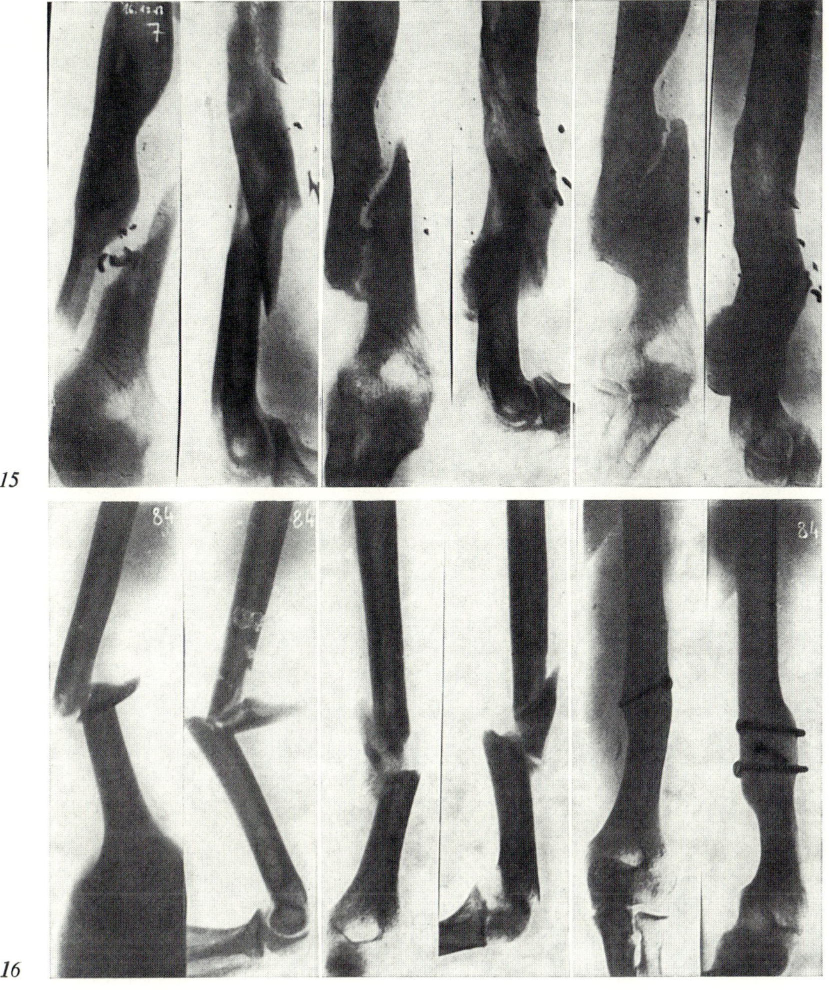

15

16

Fig. 15. Case No. 7. Miner, aged 35. Spiral fracture of the right humerus in the middle third (12 years prior to this accident he had sustained a fracture of the humerus proximal to the present site). Palm-to-shoulder cast for 31 weeks (!). Rigid non-union. At follow-up examination 11 years later the non-union had healed spontaneously. Limitations (functional): shoulder 30°, elbow 50°, pronation and supination in forearm 1/4.

Fig. 16. Case No. 84. Farmer's son, aged 19. Fracture of the left humerus at junction of middle and lowest third. Immobilisation in U-shaped splint for 12 weeks. One year after injury non-union was revealed. Step-like osteotomy and screwing. At follow-up 8 years later only terminal restriction of elbow joint. No restriction of the other arm joints.

Muscle Atrophy in the Injured Arm: In 4 Patients (7.5 %),
There Was Noted a Discrepancy
in Circumference of Arms of 1 Inch

The circumference of the arm which is used for writing, working and eating – usually the right arm – shows a surplus of more than 1 cm in general. This fact was taken into consideration in our follow-up examination. An additional discrepancy of approximately 1 in was found in 4 patients (on the upper arm as well as on the forearm, No. 7, 25, 58, 77). Two of these patients had undergone surgical treatment because of radial nerve damage.

Fracture Healing with Angulation:
In 8 Patients (15 %),
Angulation of 15–25° Was Present

In 28 patients of our follow-up series (that is in 53 % of the cases) there accurred fracture healing with angulation of more than 10°. Among them there were 8 cases with an angulation of 15–25° (No. 6, 22, 37, 41, 48, 75, 77). Varus deformity was twice as frequent than antecurvation or recurvation. The usual deformity to be found in the proximal third was antecurvation, in the middle third varus and in the distal third recurvation. Among our folluw-up patients there was only 1 case with valgus deformity. Angulation is of no importance as to function. In fractures of the distal third only a considerable angulation may slightly impair function of the elbow joint.

On the other hand, fracture healing with rotation does impair elbow function as well as pronation and supination in the forearm.

Secondary Progressive Angulation of Fracture Site
after Removal of Plaster

In our adult patients there was no change in angulation to be noted as a rule. Slight alterations were due to different planes of projection. In 2 cases, however (No. 58 and 88), there was a marked progressive angulation to be noted after removal of plaster. This illustrates the need for immobilisation until definite consolidation has occurred.

The So-Called Growing Out of Angulation in Children

In opposition to other authors we have noted that an angulation of the humeral shaft does not always grow out in children and juveniles. There were 9 children in our follow-up series. In three of them (No. 14, 76, and 85), who were 5–6 years old at the time of injury, angulation and dislocation of the fracture site 'grew out' more or less completely.

In six other cases, however (No. 12, 22, 39, 50, 66, 87), who were between 6 and 13 years at the time of injury, angulation and dislocation did not grow out completely.

Disability Pensions: 6 Cases (18 % of All Work Accidents)

33 of our follow-up patients were listed as work accidents. To six of them (18 %) a pension for permanent partial disability of 20–25 % was granted. 16 others (48 %) hat temporary pensions for less than 2 years or total indemnifications.

Non-Union: No Cases

Among our 53 follow-up patients there was no case of non-union noted. Of the 2 cases of non-union which were described in our early results, one had healed spontaneously (No. 7) and the other (No. 84), in which non-union was revealed 1 year after injury, healed after osteotomy and screwing.

Radial Nerve Palsy: 1 Case (2 %)

Seven of our 10 patients with radial nerve damage were re-examined at follow-up. There was 1 case of complete radial nerve palsy noted (No. 58), which had been treated by substitutive tendon grafting as advocated by PERTHES. In this case movement of fingers and wrist joint was limited by one half.

The other 6 patients did neither show motor impairment nor sensory deficiency at follow-up. To our regret, the patient in whom a suture of the dissected radial nerve had been carried out in 1960 did not come to follow-up.

Summary of Late Results

All 100 patients of a consecutive series of fractures of the humeral shaft, treated (mostly conservatively) in this hospital during the years 1956–1960, were invited in 1968 for re-examination. 53 attended the follow-up examination.

About half of them complained about occasional mild pain, especially during a change of weather. Limitation of motion of shoulder was rather rare. Only 3 patients ($5^1/_2$ %) showed a limitation between 30 and 50°. Three patients ($5^1/_2$ %) had a limitation of elbow between 40 and 50°. In 7 patients (13 %), pronation and supination in forearm was impaired $^1/_4$–$^1/_2$. Four patients ($7^1/_2$ %) showed a significant muscle atrophy in the injured arm. One patient (2 %) had a complete radial palsy.

These 18 functional limitations described above were found partly combined in 10 patients (19 % of our follow-up cases).

Eight patients (15 %) had fracture healing with angulation of 15–25° (mostly varus). Out of 9 children the angulation noted primarily grew out completely in 3 cases but persisted in 6 cases. Among 33 follow-up patients who had sustained work accidents, six (18 %) received final partial disability pensions ranging from 20 to 25 %.

Final Remark

The aim of this paper is neither to advocate nor to condemn methods of treatment in fractures of the humeral shaft, but simply to show what results may be expected by conservative treatment, which was the method of choice during the years 1956–1960, when this study was begun.

Nowadays we have changed our opinion in some respect and surgical treatment is more frequently applied. It would be interesting, however, to compare the final results of a group of surgically treated fractures of the humerus with a corresponding conservatively treated series.

Summary

In this statistical study 100 consecutive cases of fractures of the humeral shaft are analysed. These 100 cases were treated mainly conservatively in this hospital during the years 1956–1960 according to the principles advocated by L. BÖHLER. Early results and late results were very good in 80 % but not fully satisfactory in 20 % of the cases.

Author's address: Dr. W. HOSNER, Unfallkrankenhaus Graz, Theodor-Körner-Strasse 65, *A-8010 Graz* (Austria)

Reconstr. Surg. Traumat., vol. 14, pp. 65–74 (Karger, Basel 1974)

Fresh Fractures of the Shaft of the Humerus – Conservative or Operative Treatement?

T. RÜEDI, A. MOSHFEGH, K. M. PFEIFFER and M. ALLGÖWER

Clinic for General Surgery, Department of Surgery of the University of Basel, Basel

Contents

The best way of treating fractures of the shaft of the humerus is still much discussed. The warning of BÖHLER [1964] against approaching the humerus by open reduction should not be overheard. In his large experience of conservative treatment neither healing nor functional restitution was ever a ,problem in these fractures, but he apparently saw poor outcomes after operative treatment rather frequently. The development of good methods of internal fixation [HACKETHAL, 1961; MÜLLER, *et al.*, 1969] has on the other hand introduced tempting new possibilities which in the hand of a good surgeon may be most rewarding. Especially with the use of rigid internal fixation the immediate return to full mobility of the whole arm is of great advantage to the patient.

We agree with BÖHLER [1964] that the humerus is a well and fast healing bone where minor angulations or rotatory malalignement are compatible with full functional recovery (fig. 1). Internal fixation of the fractured humerus is, therefore, rarely done as a primary procedure,

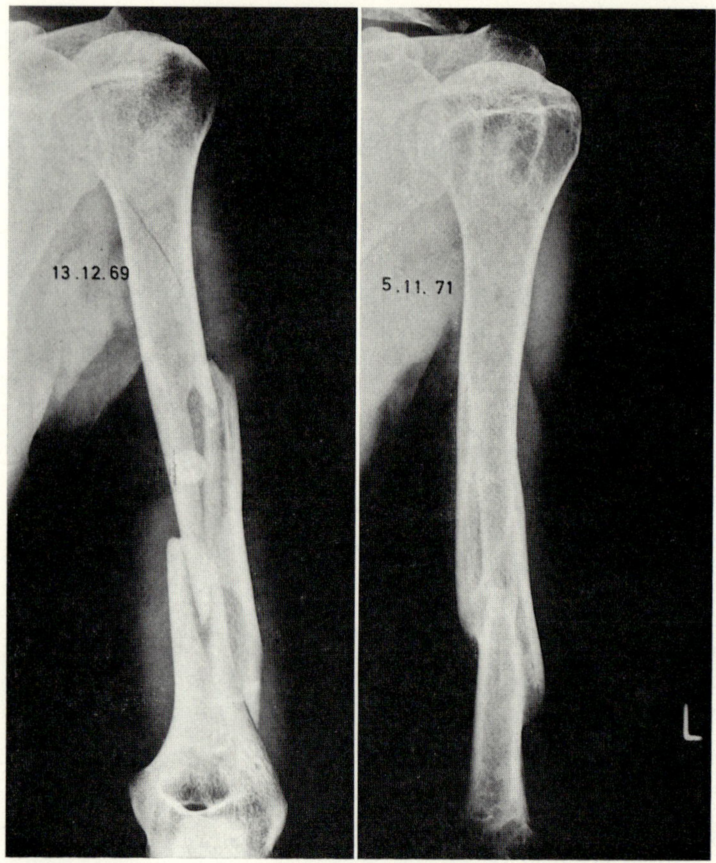

Fig. 1. Butterfly fracture of the humeral shaft, successfully treated by conservative means.

despite our different basic philosophy concerning other bones such as the forearm, the femur, and even the tibia.

Between 1968 and 1969, 52 fresh fractures of the shaft of the humerus in adult patients were treated at the University Clinic of Basle. 41 fractures or about three quarters of the cases were primarily approached by conservative means, while primary open reduction and internal fixation was performed in 11 patients as an emergency procedure and 6 times secondarily after an unsucessful conservative trial.

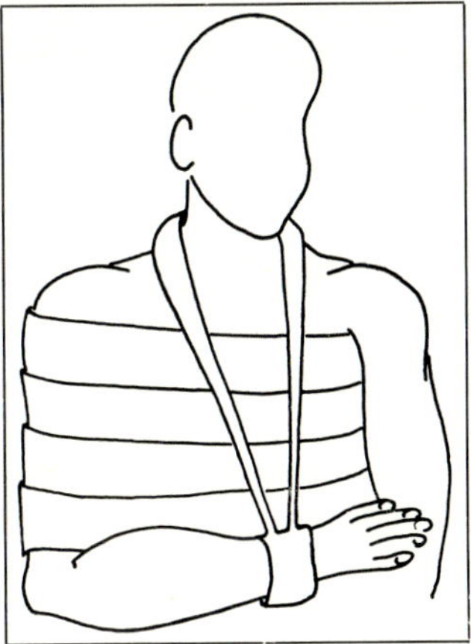

Fig. 2. Fixation of the humerus to the chest by circular bandages. The elbow is left free while the rest is supported.

Conservative Treatment

Closed fractures of the middle shaft of the humerus are in our opinion best immobilised by fixing the upper arm to the chest by large circular bandages. In contrast to the Desault splint the elbow must be left free and bent to about 80°, while the slightly supinated forearm is supported by a well-padded sling around the wrist and neck only (fig. 2). This fixation is usually sufficient as the weight of the free elbow and forearm acts in a distracting way. In oblique fractures with much shortening a hanging cast may exceptionally be applied. In dislocated short transverse fractures closed reduction under general or local anaesthesia should be attempted. The duration of fixation in the described splint varies between 4 and 6 weeks, when regular physiotherapy is started.

Pronounced obesity and large breasts may often prevent a successful reduction and adequate immobilisation of the arm in the above way, as some angulation will be almost inevitable. If in such cases after 2–3 weeks the closed treatment appears very difficult and painful, we usually feel that internal fixation is indicated. Very proximal fractures may cause similar problems of reduction and delayed healing, as the pull of the pectoralis muscle often displaces the upper fragment far medially and ventrally. Four of six secondarily operated fractures were located in the proximal third of the shaft of the humerus and did not show any sign of union within 6 weeks after fracture.

Results after Conservative Treatment

In 41 cases treated conservatively there were 6 failures, to be delt with in the next chapter. Out of 35 patients treated conservatively with success, 31 could be reviewed. Four patients could not be located any more. Complete restitution of functional integrity was regained in all instances and bony union occurred in every case. Unlike NIGST [1969], who observed a radial palsy in an earlier study in about 10 % of his cases, we did not see any such complication in the whole series of closed fractures. The incapacity for work was on average 12 weeks, although many a housewife was most probably back to cooking at an earlier date.

Operative Treatment

In the operative series (table I), we distinguish 2 groups of patients; those that were primarily operated upon and the ones that were approached secondarily after failure of conservative means.

Primary operation: Among the 11 primary operations we find 6 open fractures (table I, cases 1–6). With the exception of 1 patient all open cases displayed a concomittant nerve injury, which in the opinion of many authors [FENYÖ, 1971; SAILER *et al.*, 1969; SCHOLZE, 1970] is considered as an absolute indication for open reduction and internal fixation as well.

A 15-year-old boy (case 2) with a third degree open transverse fracture of the humerus with primary radial palsy and rupture of the biceps muscle was immediately operated upon. The radial nerve running directly across the fracture gap was severely contusioned, but not interrupted. After stable internal fixation and primary wound healing early active and passive mobilisation of the arm and hand were started and within 6 months full functional recovery of the injured limb was reestablished.

Five closed fractures of the humeral shaft (table I, cases 7–11) were also primarily approached by open reduction. Internal fixation by plating was performed between a few hours to 1 week after the accident for the following reasons: 2 patients with additional chest injuries were operated upon because any fixation of the arm to the thorax resulted in an impaired respiration. One shaft fracture was associated with a luxation of the head of the humerus, which could not be reduced by closed methods and another case presented a pathologic fracture with considerable bone loss.

The last patient (case 8, fig. 3) was hemiplegic on the contralateral side and thereby completely incapacitated. Thanks to a stable internal fixation by plating she was fully mobilised within only 10 days after the accident, walking with the aid of a cane which she carried on the operated side. No splint was used and primary union occurred without delay.

Secondary operation: In 6 patients with a closed fracture of the humeral shaft open reduction and internal fixation were performed on average 9 weeks (3–21 weeks) after the accident as a secondary procedure. The 4 cases of oblique proximal fractures that could not be reduced satisfactorily, or be kept in a reduced position by conservative means, have already been mentioned.

In a 76-year-old agitated, senile man, who did not tolerate any splint or bandages, the operative treatment was chosen for reasons of better nursing and in order to prevent skin perforation at the fully mobile fracture site. Finally the fracture of a 75-year-old woman was also operated upon as union had not occurred within 4 months after the accident.

As a means of internal fixation, plating by the ASIF technique was used in all except 2 cases. As a rule we prefer the large ASIF compression plate or the new DCP. In the wide plate the screws do not stand all in line, thus avoiding the danger of stress-fracture of the thin and brittle cortex of the humerus. Stable internal fixation by plating generally permits immediate active movement with early return to normal activity.

Two long oblique fractures of the proximal humerus were stabilized by two lag screws only, but screw fixation alone proved unsatisfactory, because they do not adequatly prevent secondary instability. Both cases produced heavy 'irritation' callus and took many weeks to unite.

The best and in our opinion the safest approach to the shaft of the humerus was found to be the dorsal exposure by HENRY [1966] with identification of the radial nerve between the heads of the triceps muscle. Without causing much damage we can expose the whole length of the shaft. The plate may – without any harm – be placed beneath the radial nerve, but care has to be taken to interpose some muscle tissue. As plates on the humerus are mostly well covered by soft tissues, they may be left in place permanently. Should removal be necessary all the same, the nerve has to be identified with utmost care.

Table I

Patient				Type of fracture	Additional lesions	Time of operation	Type of int. fix.	Complications	Results
No.	initials	age	sex						
1.	B. G.	28	♂	open, shaft R	ulnar palsy	emergency	5-hole plate	palsy recovered	good
2.	D. A.	15	♂	open, shaft L	radial palsy	emergency	5-hole plate	palsy recovered	very good
3.	H. W.	21	♂	open, shaft R	radial palsy + fract. epicondyle humeri L	emergency	7-hole plate	palsy recovered	very good
4.	K. E.	67	♂	open, shaft L	radial nerve disrupture	emergency	6-hole plate	osteitis, palsy permanent	poor
5.	R. J.	35	♂	open, shaft L	radial nerve disrupture	emergency	7-hole plate	palsy permanent	satisfactory
6.	S. R.	35	♂	open, shaft L	–	emergency	7-hole plate	refracture after new trauma	satisfactory after second op.
7.	B. E.	59	♂	closed prox. shaft R	luxation of humeral head	emergency	T-plate	† unrelated to fracture	–
8.	I. F.	61	♀	closed prox. shaft L	hemiplegia R side	emergency	7-hole plate	–	very good
9.	M. M.	49	♂	closed shaft L	thoracic lesion	2 days	7-hole plate	–	no control possible

Table I (continued)

Patient				Type of frac- ture	Addi- tional lesions	Time of opera- tion	Type of int. fix.	Com- plications	Results
No.	initials	age	sex						
10.	S. R.	45	♂	pathol. shaft L	pathol. fract.	emer- gency	8-hole plate	† from metasta- sis	–
11.	Z. D.	33	♂	closed prox. shaft R	thoracic lesion	7 days	6-hole plate	–	very good
12.	B. R.	65	♀	closed shaft L	–	after 14 weeks of con- serv. treatm.	6-hole plate	–	good
13.	B. M.	69	♂	closed prox. shaft L	–	after 3 weeks of con- serv. treatm.	9-hole plate + can- cellous autograft	–	very good
14.	C. G.	59	♂	closed prox. shaft R	–	after 8 weeks of con- serv. treatm.	1 lag screws	delayed union	very good
15.	F. O.	64	♀	closed prox. shaft L	–	after 20 weeks of con- serv. treatm.	2 lag screws	delayed union	very good
16.	M. I.	64	♀	closed prox. shaft R	–	after 5 weeks of con- serv. treatm.	10-hole plate	delayed union	good
17.	S. L.	76	♂	closed shaft L	severe cerebral arterio- sclerosis	after 2 weeks of con- serv. treatm.	7-hole plate	† 1 week postop. cardial insuff.	–

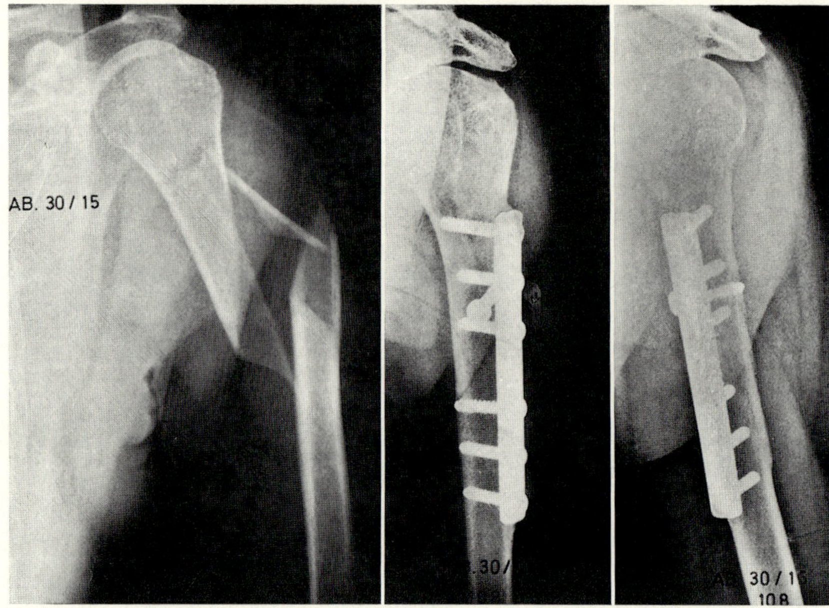

Fig. 3. Case 8: Open reduction and plate fixation of a closed fracture of the shaft of the humerus in a patient with hemiplegia of the contralateral side. Thanks to stable internal fixation the invalid patient was walking on crutches within 2 weeks.

Results after Operative Treatment

The results of 17 patients 1 year after internal fixation of the fractures of the humeral shaft may be seen in table I. Ten out of 13 cases that could be reviewed personally displayed a good or very good functional result. Three patients had died within 1 year after the accident, while 1 patient could not be reached any more. Bony union occurred in every instance, although 1 patient (case 4) with an open fracture developed an osteitis. The two unsatisfactory functional results both concern open fractures with primary damage to the radial nerve. A bridging of the nerve by suture or grafting was not performed because of infection in case 4 and in case 5 because of too large a defect. Case 6, also an open fracture, had a good result when he suffered a new trauma which caused a new fracture tearing out the plate. Elsewhere another procedure was done, but with a rather moderate outcome.

The only other complication concerns case 16, a 64-year-old woman, who produced a delayed union after a secondary operation. After introduction of a longer plate, union occurred, the final function result being good.

Discussion

In fractures of the shaft of the adult humerus again and again the question arises whether to operate or not. Against the tempting pro's, such as more comfort, immediate mobility of the arm and less pain, the serious contra's, such as the risk of anaesthesia, the risk of infection and postoperative radial palsy should not be underestimated. In view of the fast and sound funtional restitution of the fractured humerus left to spontaneous healing, we agree with BÖHLER [1964] that the majority of the closed humerus fractures should be treated conservatively.

In analysing our operative cases, on the other hand, we think that the indication for open reduction and internal fixation may be classified as absolute or relative. In our opinion an absolute indication for internal fixation is given in the case of: (a) an open fracture, especially with concomitant nerve lesions (generally as an emergency procedure); (b) in severely dislocated shaft fractures reaching into a neighbouring joint; (c) for reasons of better nursing care (polytrauma with chest injury, poly-fracture patients or very restless cases).

As relative indication are considered: (a) radial palsy in closed fractures; (b) fractures of both arms; (c) proximal shaft fractures with medial displacement of the proximal fragment.

As a stabilizing agent we usually use the new ASIF dynamic compression plate (DCP) but for transverse and short oblique fractures of the middle third of the humerus the intramedullary stacked nails by HACKETHAL [1961] constitute a very safe and elegant method of fixation, although our personal experiences with this instrumentation is limited.

Summary

Treatment of 52 consecutive cases of fresh fractures of the shaft of the humerus in the adult is reported. Three quarters of the cases were treated conservatively by simply fixing the arm to the chest. Eleven times an operative approach was chosen as an emergency procedure, including 6 open fractures with 5 concomitant nerve lesions and 5 patients in whom other circumstances called for open reduction. Six fractures were plated 3–14 weeks after the accidents because conservative treatment had failed. The comparatively better results after conservative treatment prove that uncomplicated fractures of the humeral shaft should not be primarily approached by open reduction, although the operated cases in this series constitute a negative selection.

References

Böhler, L.: Gegen die operative Behandlung von frischen Oberarmschaftbrüchen. Arch. klin. Chir. *308:* 465 (1964).

Fenyö, G.: On fractures of the shaft of the humerus. Acta chir. scand. *137:* 221 (1971).

Hackethal, K. H.: Die Bündelnagelung (Springer, Wien 1961).

Henry, A. K.: Extensile exposures; 2nd ed. (Livingstone, Edinburgh 1966).

Müller, M.; Allgöwer, M. und Willenegger, H.: Technik der operativen Frakturbehandlung (Springer, Berlin 1969).

Nigst, H.: Chirurgie der peripheren Nerven. Z. Unfallmed. Berufskr. *4:* 199 (1969).

Sailer, R.; Boettcher, J. und Kovacicek, S.: Beitrag zur Behandlung der Oberarmbrüche des Erwachsenen. Chirurg, Berlin *40:* 221 (1969).

Scholze, H.: Indikationsfehler bei der Behandlung von Oberarmschaftbrüchen. Arch. klin. Chir. *327:* 845 (1970).

Authors' address: Dr. Th. Rüedi, A. Moshfegh, Dr. K. M. Pfeiffer and Prof. Dr. M. Allgöwer, Department of Surgery of the University of Basel, Clinic for General Surgery, *CH-4000 Basel* (Switzerland)

Reconstr. Surg. Traumat., vol. 14, pp. 75–83 (Karger, Basel 1974)

The Operative Treatment of Fractures of the Shaft of the Humerus

A. Titze

Accident Hospital Graz of the General Insurance Company
(Medical Director: A. Titze), Graz

From long experience in our hospital we are convinced that in closed fractures of the shaft of the humerus conservative treatment is still the procedure of choice. We quote our earlier study of results referring to this [Hosner, 1972].

However, there are special cases in which we cannot expect satisfactory results by conservative management. The urgency for surgical operation may become evident either in the beginning or later in the course of treatment. In earlier decades, such cases of non-union, delayed union and malunion were treated by clearing out the fracture site and by wire looping. Later Küntscher nails and Rush pins were widely used. Today, we know that these procedures will not always guarantee bony union of the fracture or safe elimination of an existing pseudarthrosis.

During the last years the technique of plating as recommended by the Swiss AO group has proved to be the optimum procedure, superior to all other known methods of internal fixation. Compression plating carried out with care and precision is a safe and reliable procedure. It also has the advantage that no immobilisation in a plaster cast is required and that active exercises of all arm joints may be started immediately after operation. At the time when osteous union occurs, all arm joints have already gained free motion as a rule and full muscle strength is present.

At operation special care must be taken in order not to damage the radial nerve. The latter must be exposed with care and handled with gentleness. Its vulnerability has induced us not to remove the plates when bony union has occurred. Despite all precautions taken we have occasionally noticed transitory nerve impairment – although complete recovery occurred within weeks in all cases.

Plates provide excellent stability if they are properly applied as advocated by AO and there is no danger of plate loosening, which of course would impair the consolidation of the fracture. We do not use plates shorter than such with seven holes and we prefer even longer ones with eight to ten holes. In doubt always a longer plate is recommended.

So far we have not seen a wound infection after plating of a humeral fracture.

Pseudarthrosis with abundant callous of connective tissue is treated by compression only, without the callous being removed. The plate is always fixed on the convex side. In non-union with inactive atrophic bone and sclerotic fracture zones, decortication is carried out and a cancellous bone graft is applied at the time of plating.

At our hospital we have established the following indications for plating in fractures of the humeral shaft:

1. Primary Ostheosynthesis

(a) Open fractures with widely exposed fracture site or radial nerve palsy.

(b) Fractures on the level middle distal third with radial palsy. Here the nerve lies close to the bone and is susceptible to crushing between the fracture fragments. In these cases an exploration of the nerve is carried out and the fracture is stabilised by plating.

(c) Polytraumatisised patients with humeral fractures. Here often osteosynthesis is advisable to facilitate nursing. The same applies to patients with cerebral trauma, especially when they have spasms. Exact immobilisation of the arm is then often only practicable by internal fixation.

2. Secondary Ostheosynthesis

(a) Delayed union or impending non-union (fig. 1–4).

(b) Refractures of the humerus. Because in these cases a high percentage of impaired fracture-healing is noted (fig. 5, 6).

(c) Non-union (fig. 7, 8).

(d) If previous operations have failed and non-union is present (fig. 9, 10).

Excellent results may be expected by compression plating if the guiding principles as laid down by the Swiss AO group are observed: i. e. knowledge of bio-mechanical laws, perfect technique of plating, high standard of surgery and uneventful wound healing, postoperative care without immobilisation and early beginning with active exercises. If full attention is paid to these points the technique of compression plating will prove to be a safe and reliable procedure, especially in those cases in which conservative treatment has failed.

Nonetheless, we are convinced that the vast majority of closed fractures of the humeral shaft should be treated now as before conservatively because of the fact that 90 % of closed fractures will unite by this treatment within 6–10 weeks in good position and without any risk.

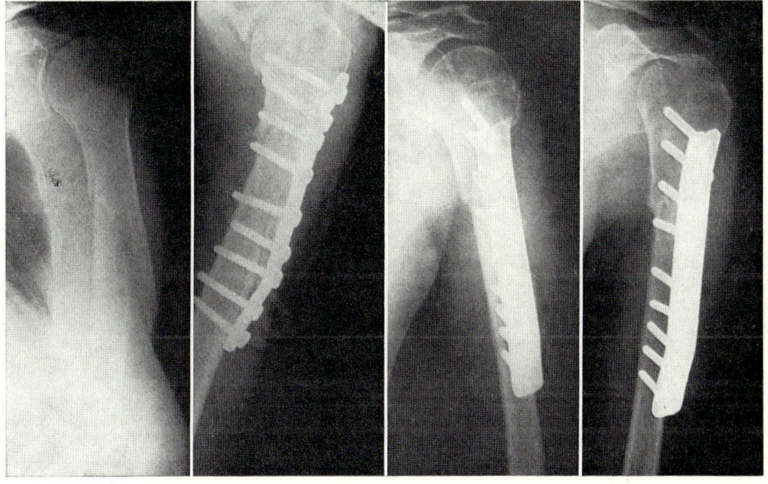

Fig. 1. Record No. 05102/71. H. M., a 65-year-old female shopkeeper, fell from a ladder on 10-3-1971 and sustained a fracture of the left humerus and accessory injuries. The fracture was treated conservatively in an outward hospital by an O-shaped plaster splint for six weeks. A few days after removal of plaster she fell again on her left arm and during the following weeks she complained about pains in the arm. Because of increasing angulation and instability of the fracture we carried out compression-plating on 26-5-1971. Three months later only slight limitation of shoulder movement was present and full function in all other arm joints.

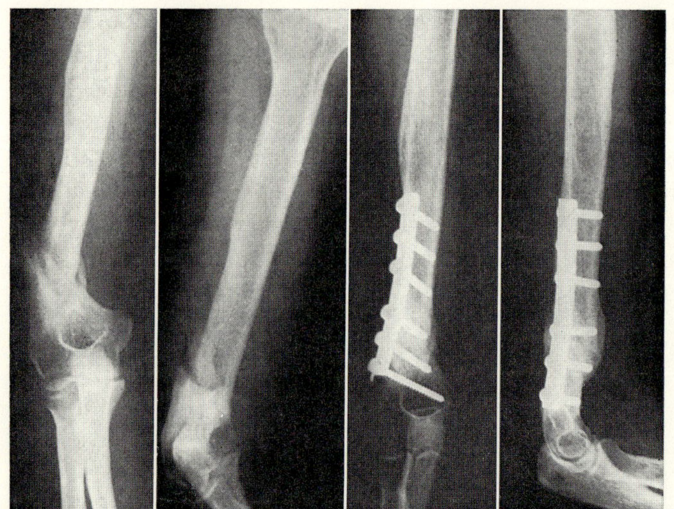

2

3

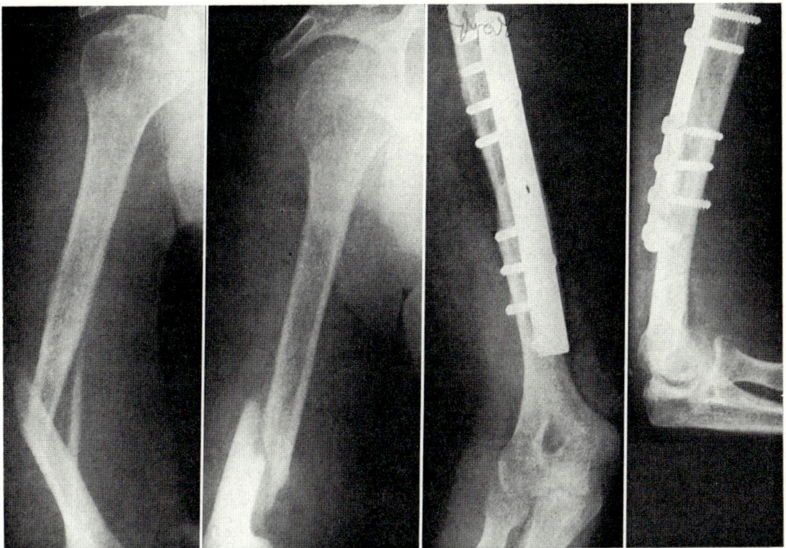

4

Fig. 2. Record No. 23867/71. C. K., a 50-year-old female employee, was injured in a road accident and sustained a fracture of the right humerus. Se was admitted to an outward hospital, where her fracture was immobilised by palm-to-shoulder plaster cast for 14 weeks. On the day that the plaster was removed, marked angulation and instability of the fracture was present. Because of this we carried out open reduction and plating. Transitory radial nerve impairment was noted after operation which subsided completely after several months. Otherwise the post-operative course has been uneventful.

Fig. 3. Record No. 02881/69. A. I., a mechanic aged 24, fell from a ladder on 17-9-1968 and sustained a fracture of the right humerus which was treated conservatively in an outward hospital. When the plaster cast was revomed 3½ months later, delayed union was noted. On 11-2-1969 we carried out compression-plating. In July 1969 radiographs showed loosening of the plate and non-union still present. Because of this we had to change the plate on 24-7-1969. The further course was uneventful. Follow-up examination showed full function in all arm-joints and solid union.

Fig. 4. Record No. 15355/70. A. H., a typist aged 49, was injured abroad in a road accident on 18-7-1970 and sustained a fracture of the right humerus. Primary treatment: Desault's plaster cast. Four months later the plaster was removed and delayed union was found. After a few days skin care, we performed compression plating combined with cancellous bone grafting. Uneventful recovery. Two months after operation, only 20° lack of extension in the elbow was noted, but full function in all other arm joints.

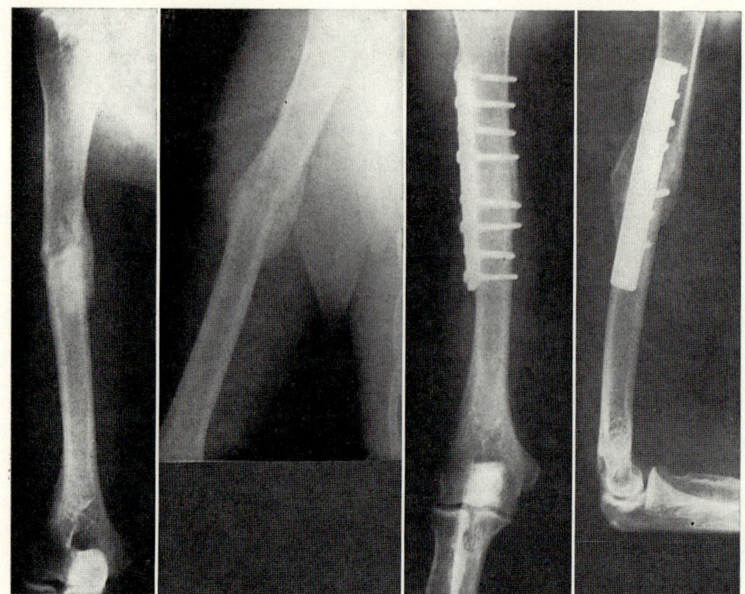

5

6

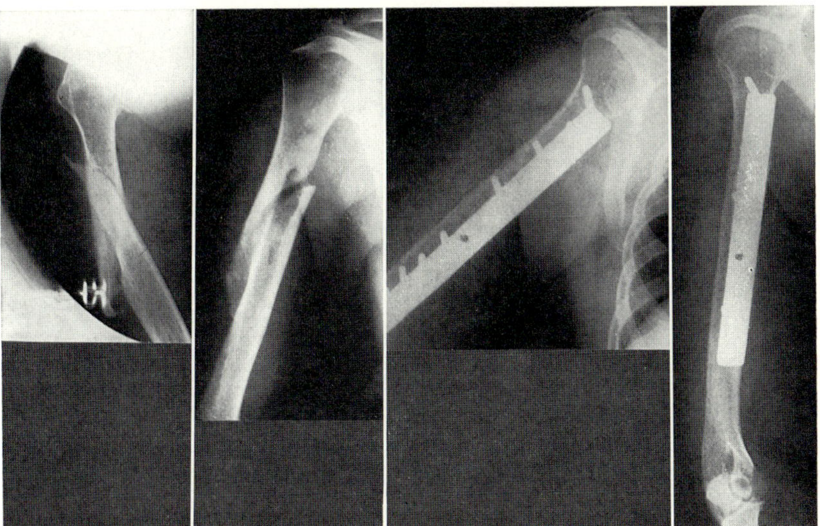

7

Fig. 5. Record No. 00813/71. F. W., a road-man aged 60, fell to the ground on an icy road on 11-1-1971 and refractured his right humerus (previous fracture on same level in August 1970). Three days after admission to our hospital we carried out compression plating. Further uneventful course. Follow-up in November 1971 showed no limitation in arm joints.

Fig. 6. Record No. 13250/69. I. H., an assistant foreman aged 28, was injured in a road accident on 30-5-1968. He sustained many injuries including a rupture of the liver, multiple rib fractures and a fracture of the right humerus. Primary treatment was carried out in an outward hospital, where the humeral fracture was stabilised by wire-looping and plating. When we saw the patient in June 1969 non-union (after refracture) was evident. Because of this we removed all metal implantations and cleared out the pseudarthrosis. After this compression plating was performed. At follow-up in November 1969 the patient had full range of shoulder movement and full range of elbow movement. Radiographs showed bony union.

Fig. 7. Record No. 23111/69. H. K., a pensioner aged 54, was injured in a road accident on 2-11-1968. Primary treatment in an outward hospital consisted of immobilisation of the humeral fracture by palm-to-shoulder plaster. We saw the patient one year later, when non-union was evident. We carried out open reduction after removing the soft callous and we stabilised the fracture by a plate. Uneventful recovery. At follow-up there was only found terminal restriction of movement in the arm joints.

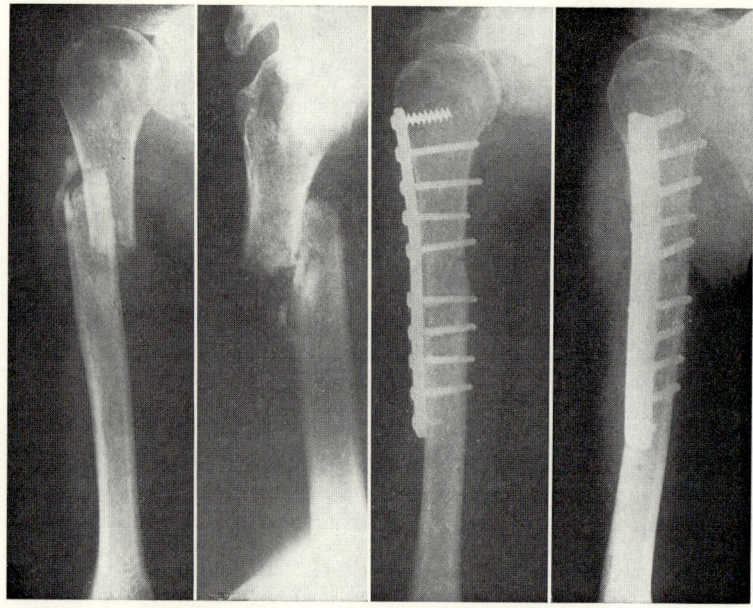

Fig. 8. Record No. 25739/70. A. S., a miner aged 48, sustained multiple injuries in a motorbike accident on 12-6-1970. A palm-to-shoulder cast was applied in an outward hospital and the plaster was removed four and a half months later. Non-union was present in December 1970, when the patient was admitted to our hospital. We performed open reduction and compression-plating. At follow-up examination two months later free range of motion in all arm joints was found.

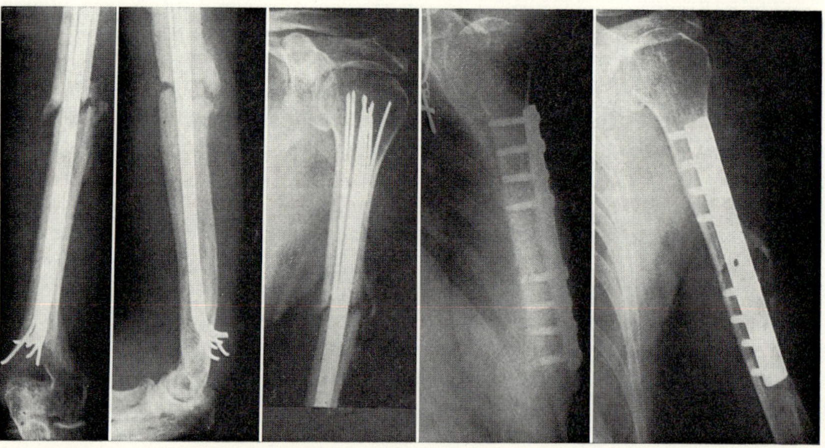

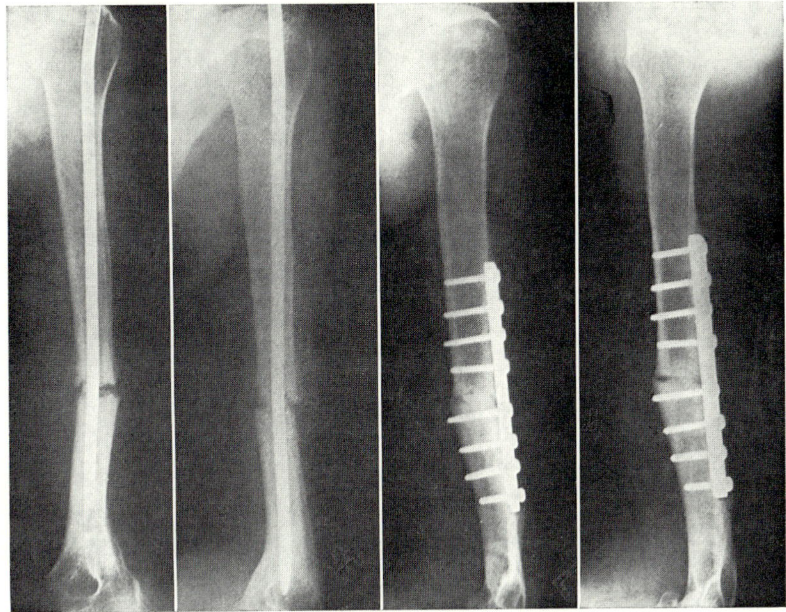

Fig. 9. Record No. 11512/70. F. T., a 57-year-old labourer, was run over by a motor car on 8-12-1969 on a street-crossing and sustained a fracture of the left humerus. He was admitted to an outward hospital, where the fracture was stabilised by intramedullary wire pins and by a plaster cast. We saw the patient six months later, when non-union was present. We removed the wire pins and carried out compression plating. The patient resumed work eight weeks after operation. At follow-up in November 1970 full function in all arm joints was noted.

Fig. 10. Record No. 8322/69. O. H., a 37-year-old truck driver, was injured in a street accident on 11-11-1968, when he sustained an open fracture of the left humerus. He also had multiple fractures of ribs and other injuries. He was admitted to an outward hospital where intramedullary nailing of the humerus was performed. When we saw the patient five months later non-union was evident. Because of this we removed the nail and carried out compression plating. Transitory radial nerve impairment was noted after operation, which subsided completely after several weeks. At follow-up examination in December 1969 good function in all arm joints was noted.

Author's address: Univ.-Doz. Dr. ALOIS TITZE, Theodor-Körner-Strasse 65, A-8010 Graz (Austria)

Reconstr. Surg. Traumat., vol. 14, pp. 84–106 (Karger, Basel 1974)

Plastic and Reconstructive Surgery in Trauma

K. WINTSCH and E. PAMPURIK

Plastic Surgery Unit, Surgical Clinic (Chief Surgeon: Prof. F. DEUCHER),
Kantonsspital, Aarau

Contents

Introduction (by Dr. DEUCHER, Chief Surgeon)

For many years we have emphasised that a surgical clinic of the size
of the clinic in Aarau (with more than 1,000 accident inpatients, more
than 10,000 outpatient consultations and with approximately 2,000 ambulatory operations per year) should have a specialist in plastic and reconstructive surgery. It was not only difficult to convince the authorities,
even medical doctors from different sections showed little understanding.
According to them a general surgeon should be able to treat all kinds of
injuries. They believed that for the rest a plastic and reconstructive surgeon would only be occupied with aesthetic surgery for which there was
no need in a general surgical clinic.

My conviction has always been that we must have specialists in leading positions for all those problems where the general surgeon cannot
(beside his other tasks) acquire enough experience and enough knowledge.
In addition to other specialists a full-time plastic surgeon has now been in
a leading position in our department for $1^{1}/_{2}$ years.

In the short time of his activity in our clinic he was able to prove, together with his co-worker, how important their cooperation was for the treatment of casualties. As a matter of fact, this cooperation has become indispensable for us.

For these reasons I am surprised that not only hospitals like ours, but even university hospitals think that they can manage without specialists for plastic and reconstructive surgery. Our personal experience has confirmed my opinion, that these specialists must be integrated into each hospital in which a great number of trauma casualties has to be treated daily.

From this will benefit: (a) the patients, who are treated better, rehabilitated sooner and who will be disabled less frequently or to a smaller extent; (b) those who have to bear the expenses, like insurance companies, as there is no doubt that the initial treatment by a skilled specialist reduces the number of secondary procedures; (c) the specialists themselves, because they increase their experience by treating fresh injuries; (d) the residents of the surgical clinic, who are taught and supervised in basic techniques of plastic and reconstructive surgery, and finally (e) the hospital, because with the number of special services its reputation increases.

General Statements

The majority of plastic surgery procedures are time-consuming. These operations are generally not of vital importance and sometimes even not of functional value. For these reasons in times when many casualties are arriving at an emergency station at the same time the plastic surgery cases may be considered less important and there is the temptation to have them treated by junior members of the staff. The treatments are then performed with lack of time and lack of knowledge. The fate of many of these injuries greatly depends on the quality of the initial treatment. These operations need a specially fine operation technique, skill and knowledge in skin transplantation procedures and skin flaps and a great deal of patience.

Often parts of exposed bones and other valuable tissues may be saved with the use of flaps or other procedures. The plan for later reconstruction may influence the initial repair. In such a way time can be saved.

So for many accident patients it means an important improvement when a plastic surgery team is attached to a clinic treating casualties. In a hospital with a separate clinic for plastic and reconstructive surgery in-

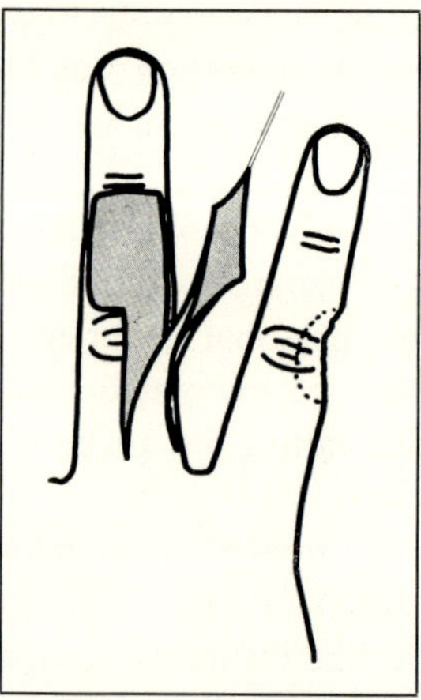

Fig. 1. The flag flap may be used for similar purpouses as a cross finger flap. It can reach almost any region of the neighbouring finger.

juries of the face and the hand may be brought directly to this department and teamwork will be reserved for cases having multiple injuries or injuries that have to be treated by both the traumatic or general surgeon and the plastic surgeon. However, a plastic surgeon or a plastic surgery team is often part of a general or traumatic surgical clinic.

Under these conditions the minor plastic surgery problems are handled by the trauma staff. For these cases the plastic surgeon may give his advice if asked for. He also takes the responsibility for the education of junior members of the surgical clinic in his field. At times when many casualties are taking all the time of the emergency team the plastic surgeon will share the burden by taking care even of minor cases in his speciality.

In the following 3 chapters we shall show examples of casualties that benefit when a plastic surgery team is attached to a clinic taking care of trauma patients. The chapters are: (1) plastic and reconstructive surgery in fresh trauma cases; (2) early reconstruction programmes in trauma; (3) skin flaps as secondary procedures in trauma.

1. Plastic and Reconstructive Surgery in Fresh Injuries

If, in soft tissue defects, joints, bones or tendons are exposed we should cover them by living tissue and provide them with the patient's own blood supply. This should be done without delay in order to avoid necrosis of these valuable structures. Different kinds of pedicled skin flaps serve this purpose.

In a finger such a defect may be covered by a simple crossfinger flap. Finger parts that cannot be reached by a cross finger flap are better treated with the so-called flag flap (fig. 1). This flap makes use of the same soft tissue of the dorsal part of the middle phalanx as a cross finger flap. A long mobile pedicle from the dorsum of the proximal phalanx enables it to reach almost any region of any finger.

In a degloving injury of the thumb the exposed phalanx may be saved by covering it with a tubed flap. This flap will be part of the later reconstruction. The aesthetic result is best if it is taken from the other arm as a cross arm flap (fig. 2). In a later operation sensibility has to be provided to this reconstructed thumb. This is performed with a neurovascular island flap (fig. 4).

From an amputated digit parts may be used directly or may be buried subcutaneously for later use. Nerves may be used as free grafts in nerve defects of other injured fingers. Parts of bones that have been implanted subcutaneously may later be included in tubed flaps for finger reconstruction. The site where these bones are implanted is the region of the planned flap. Exact implantation allows in a later operation easy attachment to the amputation stump. Nerves may also be implanted for later use. In a case of an amputated thumb, for example, the bone of the thumb was directly fixed to the bone of the stump, the nerves with their terminal pulp branches were sutured to the nerve endings in the stump and all this was covered by a tubed flap. The final result was a thumb with protective sensibility. No further corrections were asked for.

In major facial injuries real tissue defects are rare, exept in high velocity injuries like shotgun wounds. This means that in many of these injuries an almost perfect primary repair is possible. If primary treatment of the same wounds is inadequately performed later corrections are often difficult and will rarely lead to the same good result. In major injuries of the face we must always look for injuries of special structures. Dissections of branches of the facial nerve, lacerations of the lacrimal duct and of the parotic duct are important. Immediate repair of these structures is important. Figure 6 shows an example: In a car accident half of the nose and upper lip, the left lower eyelid and part of the zygomatic bone were torn off, remaining attached laterally. Immediate repair consisted of scraping the open maxillary sinus, attaching the zygomatic bone with wire to

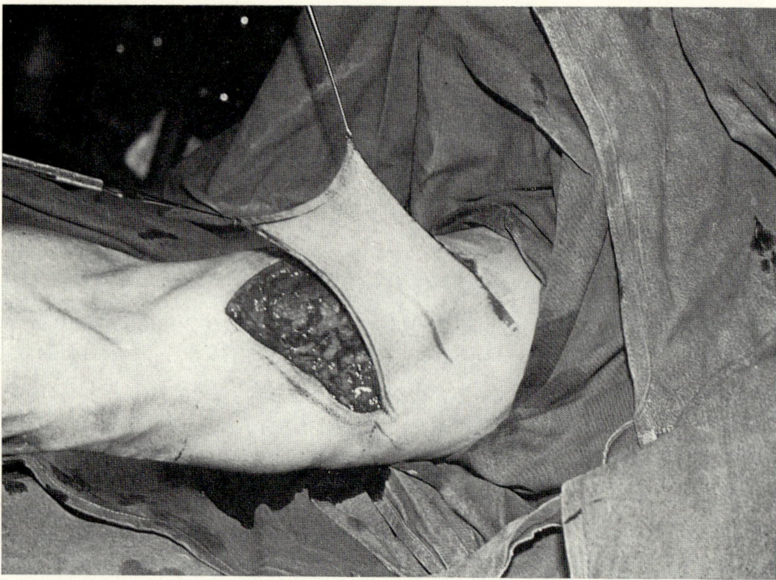

Fig. 2. A cross arm flap is raised on the right arm to cover the exposed proximal phalanx of the left thumb in a degloving injury.

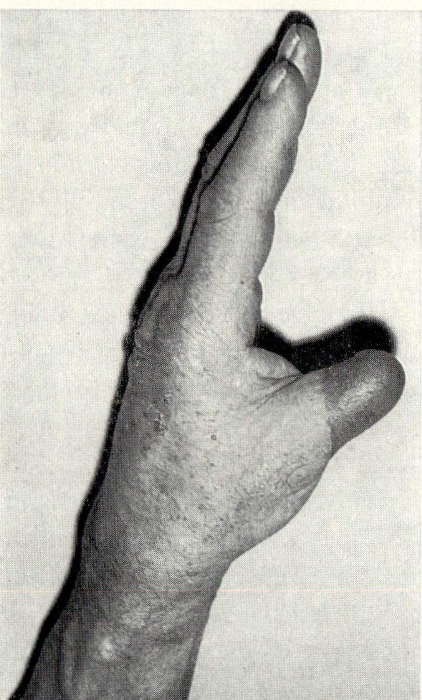

Fig. 3. In this way the whole length of the exposed bones can be saved.

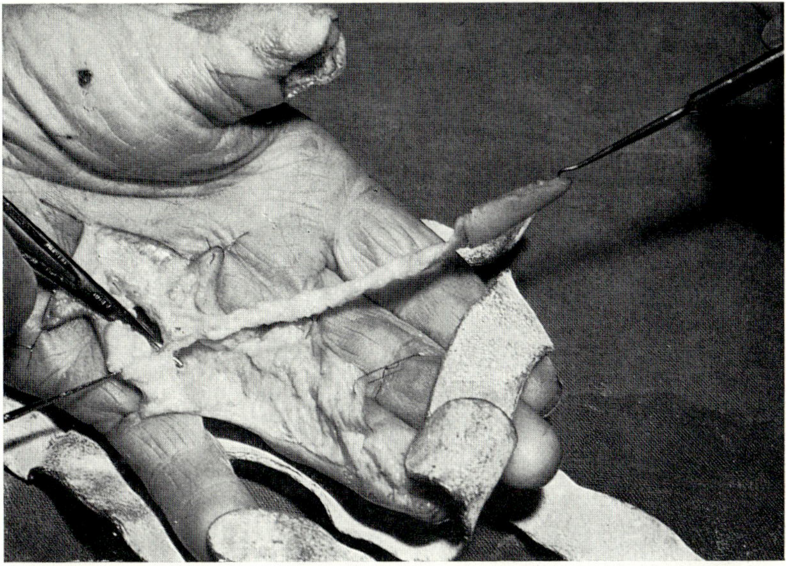

Fig. 4. Sensibility is provided to this thumb with a neurovascular island flap from the ulnar side of the ring finger.

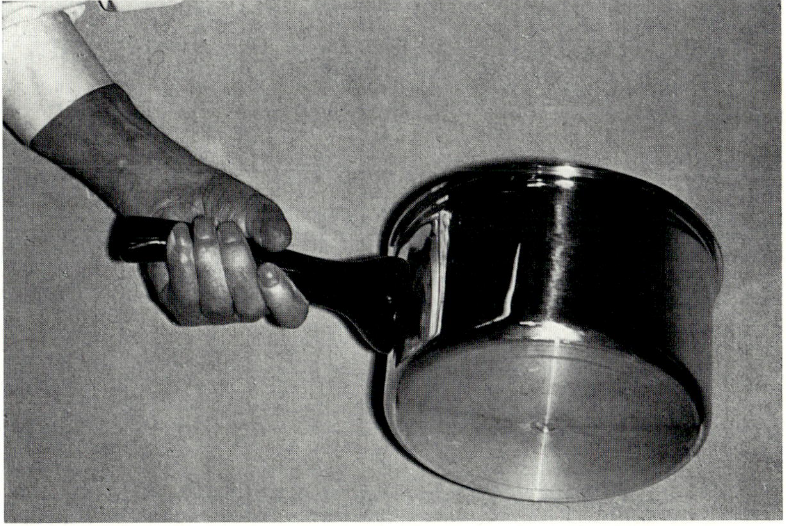

Fig. 5. Good functioning of the reconstructed thumb. The neurovascular island is in the appropriate place for grasp.

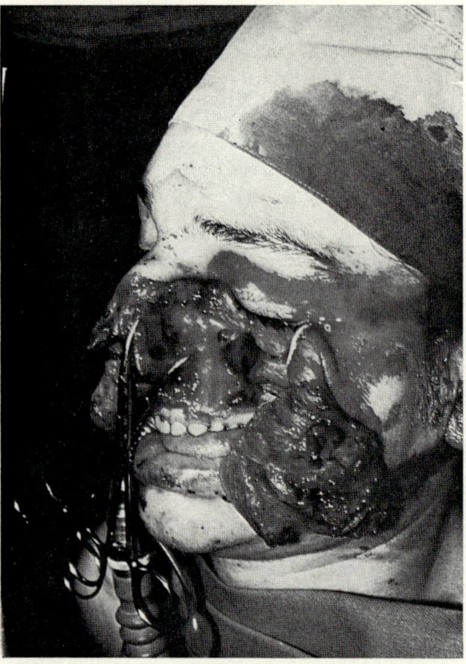

Fig. 6a. In a car accident the nose and left side of the midface has been avulsed and hangs like a flap to the left side. The maxillary sinus is open.

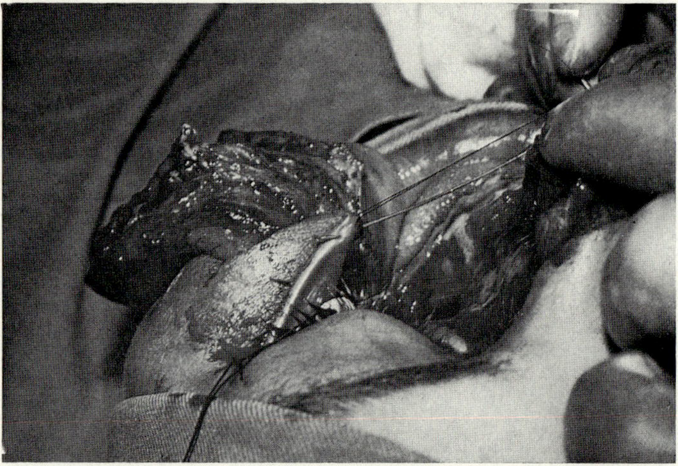

Fig. 6b. The lower eyelid has been torn off at its nasel side. A 4–0 nylon thread is passed through the punctum and the lower lacrimal duct. This thread will be used for internal splinting of the lacrimal duct.

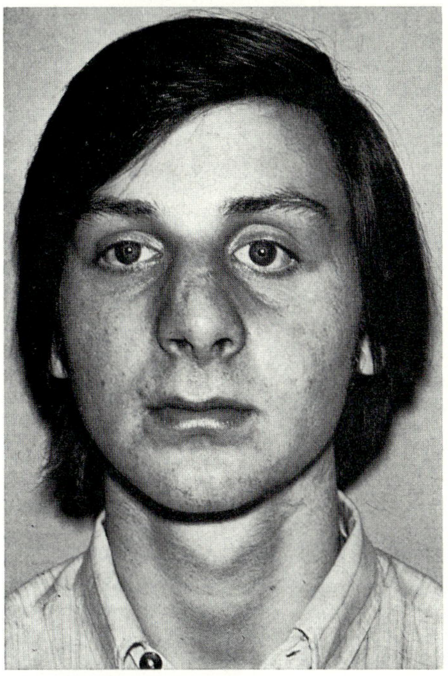

Fig. 6c. Result after primary repair. Only minor corrections will be necessary.

the maxilla, repair of the torn lower lacrimal duct (fig. 6b) and closure of all wounds. The result (fig. 6c) was such that only minor scar corrections were necessary after 6 months.

In severe hand injuries we generally save as much of viable parts as possible. The policy used to be to attempt at the first stage skin coverage of all the wounds and repair of fractures only. If necessary this was achieved with the aid of skin grafts or skin flaps. Today there is a tendency to repair more during the emergency operation. Together with the skin we tend to repair the nerves and even the tendons primarily. Bone defects are often bridged by grafts during primary repair. In severe injuries we may of course only do so if these repairs can be done without further incisions and without danger for the viable damaged tissues. A right hand and forearm after a band saw injury is shown (fig. 7). Multiple wounds with open fractures with a defect of the distal ulna, an

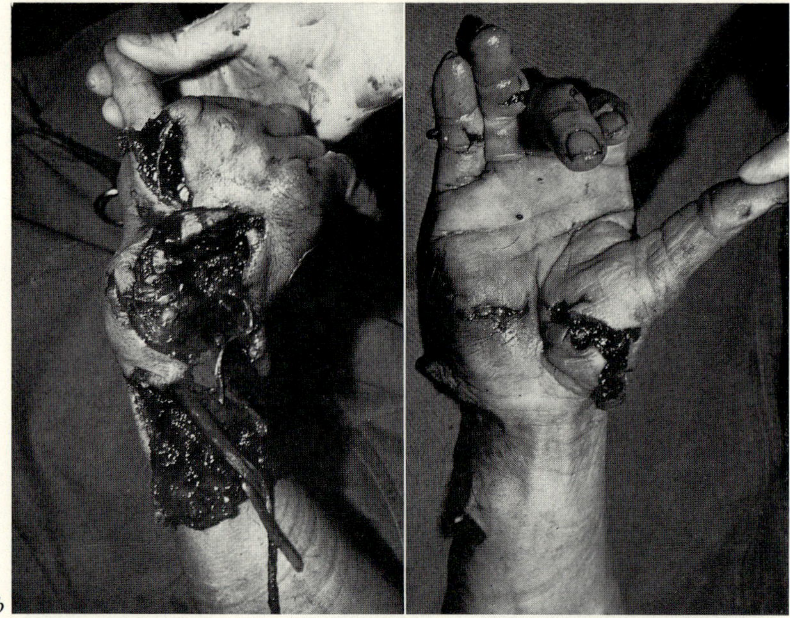

7a, b

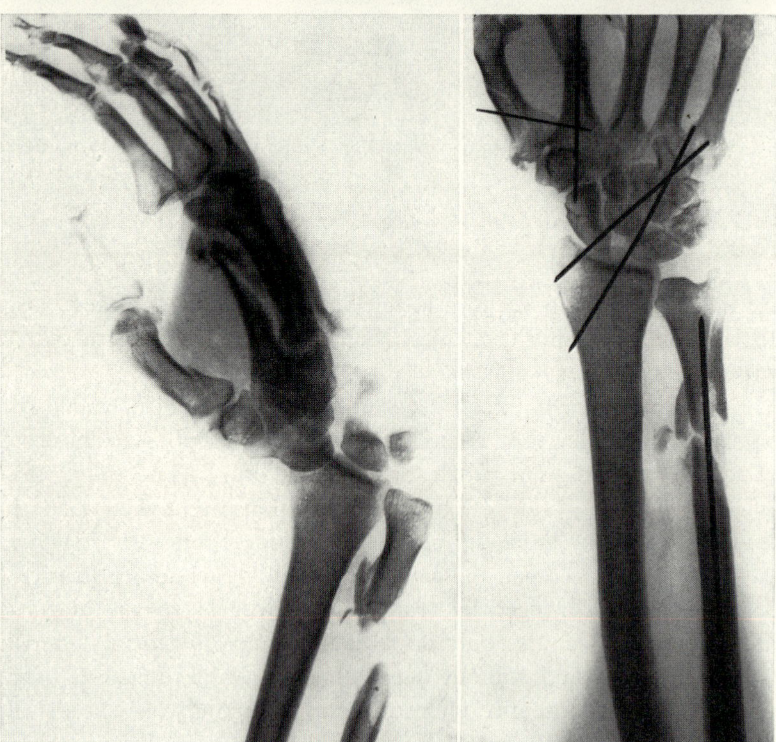

7c, d

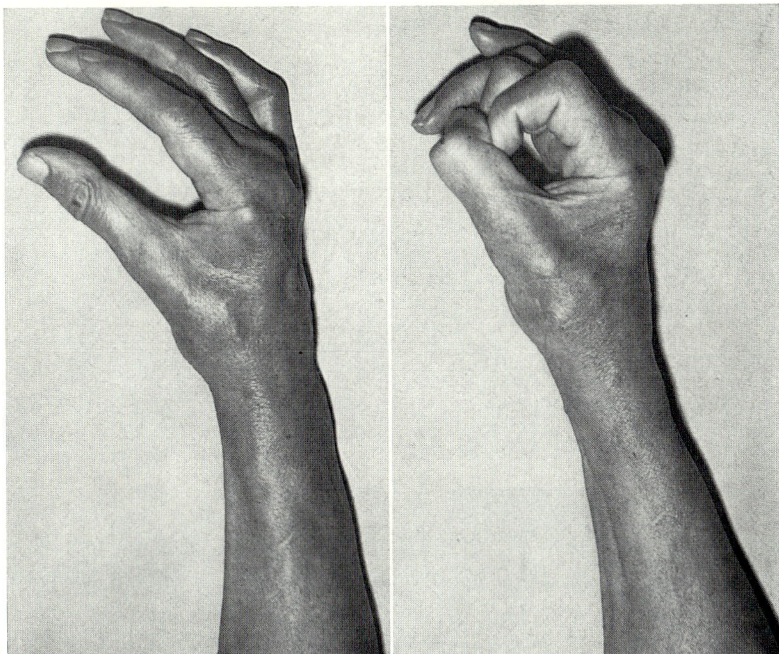

8a, b

Fig. 7a, b. A circle saw injury.

Fig. 7c. X-Ray picture of the injured hand and forearm.

Fig. 7d. X-Ray showing stabilisation of the fractures. Note that the bone gap in the ulna is bridged by a graft of spongiotic bone.

Fig. 8. Primary result after healing of the fractures: *a* active extension of the fingers; *b* flexion. Further improvement will be achieved after tenolysis of extensor tendons and capsulectomy of metacarpophalangeal joints.

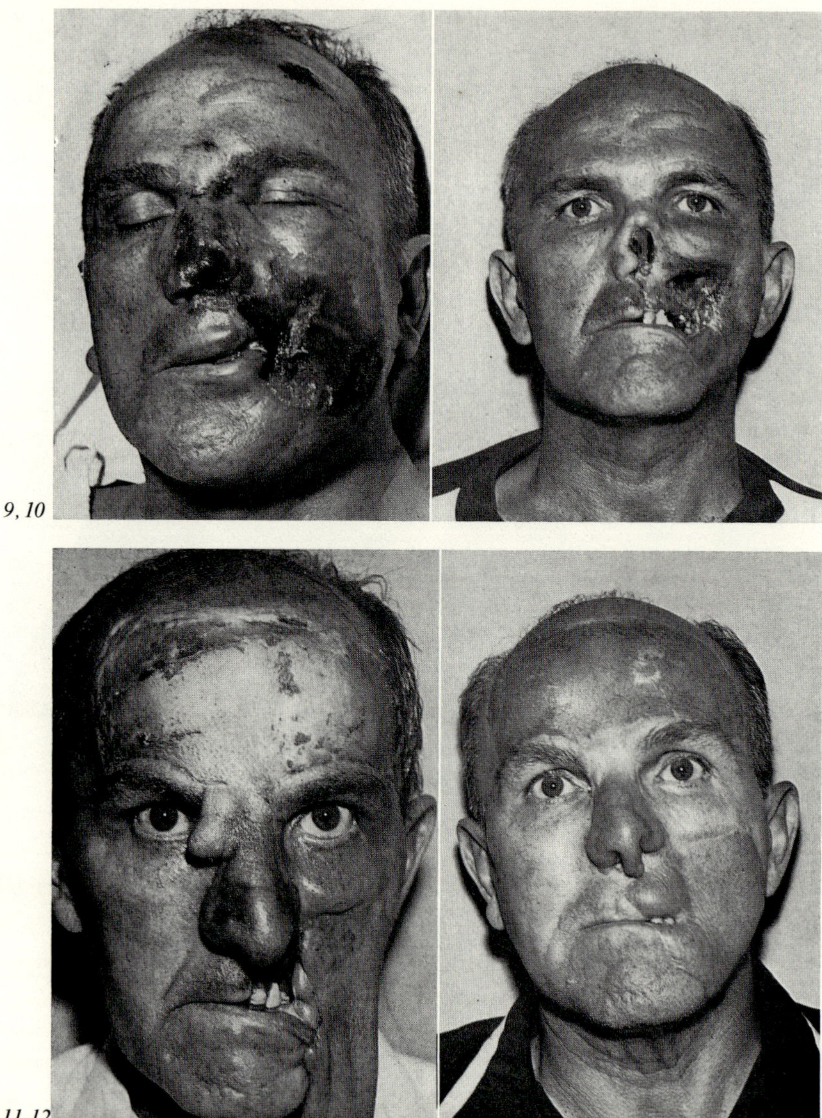

Fig. 9. A deep electric burn of the face.

Fig. 10. After debridement and skin grafting.

Fig. 11. The right half of the frontal skin was turned down as a so-called 'Indian flap' to reconstruct the nose. Simultaneous bone grafting was performed for the nose with a rib. The left half of the frontal skin was turned in as a flap on a subcutaneous pedicle to provide the bucal layer of the cheek. A deltopectoral flap was used for the outside of the cheek.

Fig. 12. Result after dissection of the deltopectoral flap.

open luxation of the wrist joint with exposed and ruptured extensor tendons, open fractures of index, ring and little fingers and dissection of the ulnar nerve at two levels were present. Primary repair consisted of reduction and Kirschner wiring of all fractures and of the luxation of the wrist. Insertion of a graft of spongitic bone in the ulna defect, primary nerve and tendon suturing. The wounds were closed. At the dorsum of the hand a skin defect was covered with a split skin graft. The result after 8 weeks was such (fig. 8) that fair function can be expected after capsulotomy of the m. p. joints of ring and little fingers and after tenolysis of the extensor tendons. In these cases the repair as such is not the only difficult part of the work. The correct judgement of what can and what cannot be done may be even more important for the fate of the injury.

2. Early Reconstruction Programmes in Trauma

An early programme for reconstruction in difficult cases saves time. With a plastic surgery team 'in the house' the programme starts immediately. This is especially important in burn patients. The history of modern medicine has proved that especially in this field cooperation of both specialities is extremely valuable. An example may show how time can be saved in an early reconstruction programme.

A 56-year-old man had a deep electric burn of the nose (fig. 9) the left half of the upper lip and the left cheek. 14 days after the injury a well-defined necrosis was present and debridement was performed. The major part of the nose, the left half of the upper lip, the left cheek and part of the zygomatic bone had to be removed. The maxillary sinus was open. The wounds were treated with physiological saline solution and split skin grafting was performed, 25 days after the injury (fig. 10).

27 days later in a major operation the nose was reconstructed with the so-called Indian frontal flap combined with primary bone grafting (the cantilever procedure of Millard). The bucal side of the cheek was repaired with the left side of the frontal skin as a subcutaneously pedicled skin flap. A deltopectoral flap was used to cover the outside of the cheek (fig. 11). Three weeks later the pedicle of the deltopectoral flap was dissected. After this the main reconstruction was ended. From then on the patient's appearance allowed him to be seen in public. He was discharged from the hospital. Further corrections were either done as an outpatient or with short stays in hospital (fig. 12).

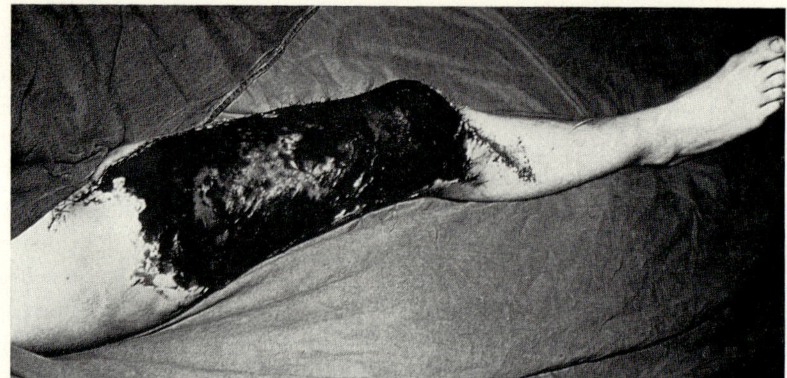

13

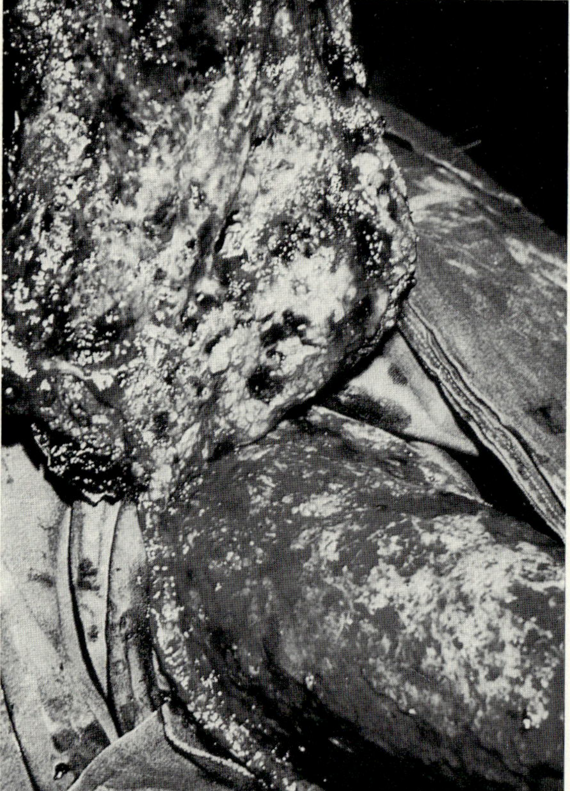

14

Fig. 13. In this case of an avulsion injury the avulsed skin flap has been sutured back without removal of the damaged subcutaneous tissue. As a result almost the total avulsed skin has become necrotic.

Fig. 14. In the upper left corner of the picture the necrotic skin with its subcutaneous tissue, which has acted like a barrier. In the lower right corner the exposed fascia.

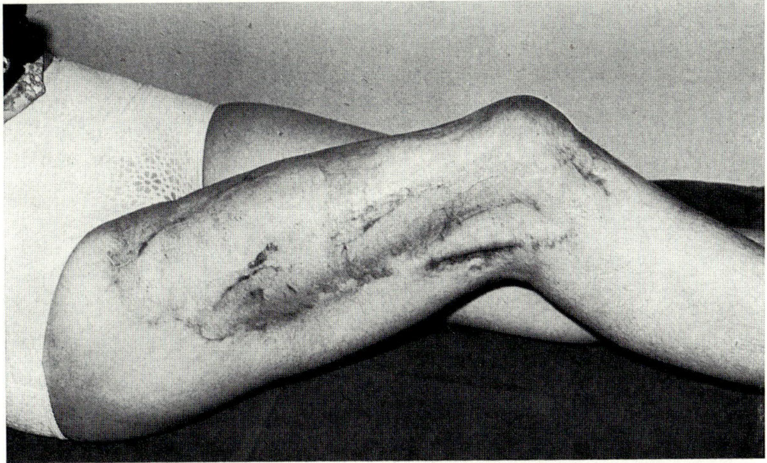

Fig. 15. After excision of the necrosed skin and split skin grafting, healing occurred within 10 days with a satisfactory functional and aesthetic result.

3. Skin Flaps as Secondary Procedures in Trauma

In secondary repair after trauma the plastic surgeon often has the task to repair extensive soft tissue defects or losses of other structures like nerves, tendons or bones.

The avulsion or degloving injury is a typical example of this kind. With mechanical progress and increase of traffic this kind of injury has become quite frequent and may happen to any exposed part of the body. From the head, ears or from the limbs the more mobile skin with the subcutaneous tissue is torn off from the stable immobile fascia or galea underneath and is damaged more or less extensively. It remains attached to the body on one side like a flap. If this avulsion flap is simply sutured back, the damaged subcutaneous tissue will act like a barrier (fig. 13 and 14) and mostly the whole flap will become necrotic. Healing will be delayed essentially. The result may be stiffness of the nearby joints causing even more time loss for rehabilitation of movement. Only if the subcutaneous tissue is completely removed from the avulsed flap the skin has the possibility to survive like a full thickness skin graft. If by incorrect treatment the avulsed skin has become necrotic it will be replaced by split skin grafts (fig. 15).

In some regions (e. g. when joints are exposed) the defects have to be convered by flaps. In primary judgement of the viability of the avulsed

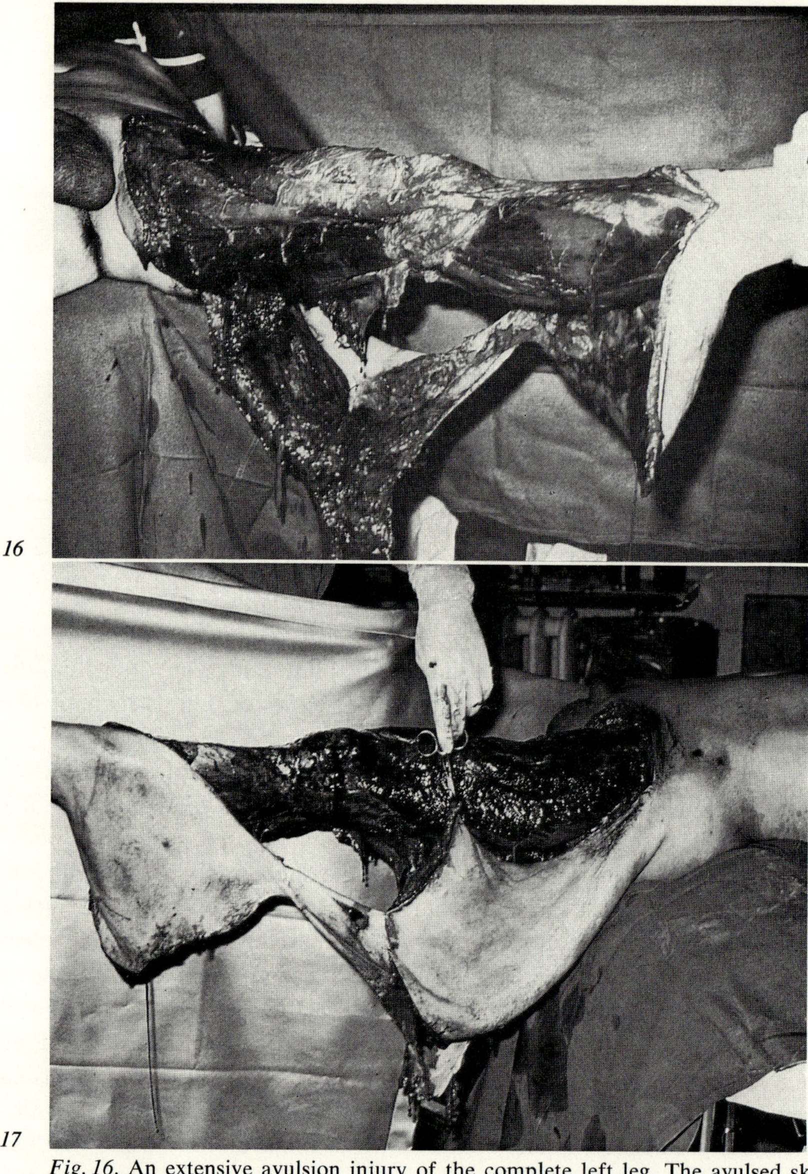

Fig. 16. An extensive avulsion injury of the complete left leg. The avulsed skin is hanging down.

Fig. 17. Vital staining by intravenous administration of Disulphin-blue of tempest was used to evaluate which parts of the avulsion flaps had an adequate blood supply. After removal of the subcutaneous tissue the skin was sutured back. Only 25 % of the avulsed skin became necrotic.

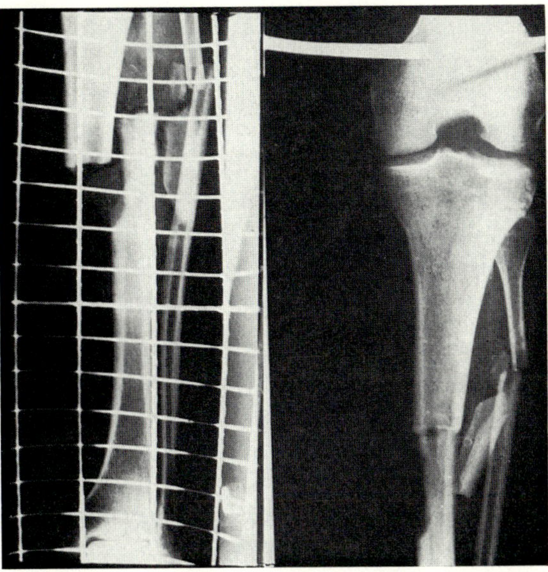

Fig. 18. Open fracture of the tibia with soft tissue defect. On the left side the primary condition. To the right after reduction. After extensive necrosis of soft tissues partial exposure of the infected bone. The infected bone ends will be excised. There will be a demand for soft tissue transplantation and subsequent bone grafting.

skin flap we have found the intravenous vital staining to be very useful (fig. 16 and 17).

If soft tissue defects are combined with fractures it is most important to cover the fractured bone with viable tissue. (fig. 18). In late cases with exposed fractures we have to provide a sufficient amount of tissue with a good blood supply in order to create favourable conditions for later bone grafting. Sometimes the local conditions are such that a local flap or a cross leg flap are adequate to solve the problem. Often, however, larger parts of tissue and bone are necrotic and more distant, larger flaps are necessary. Transport of this flap may be started together with early operations for the wound (fig. 19 and 20). It is essential to plan the flap large enough. We have to take in account that complications during flap transport may lead to minor necrosis with partial loss of the flap material. In such a way an excess of tissue will allow easy modelling of the flap and provide optimal conditions for further operations (fig. 21 and 22).

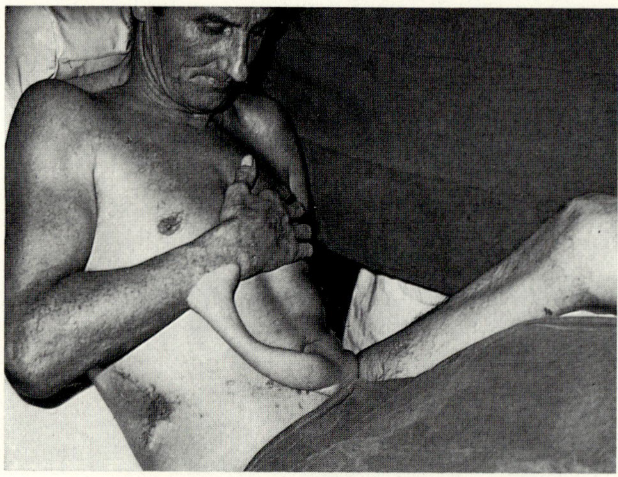

Fig. 19. During early treatment of the open fracture a large tube pedicled flap is constructed on the abdomen. It is transported by the right arm.

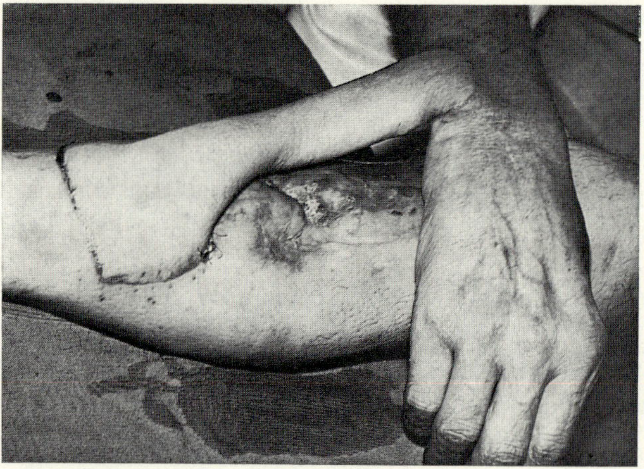

Fig. 20. The flap is brought down to the damaged leg.

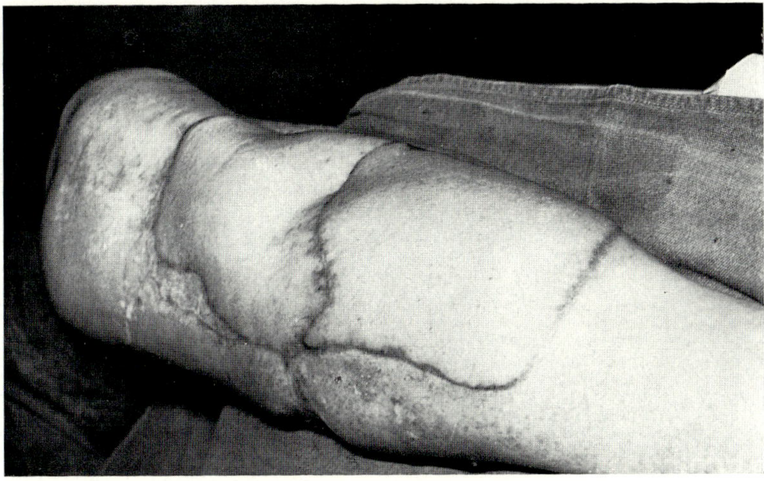

Fig. 21. Meanwhile the osteomyelitis has healed and now the bone defect underneath the flap is ready for bone grafting.

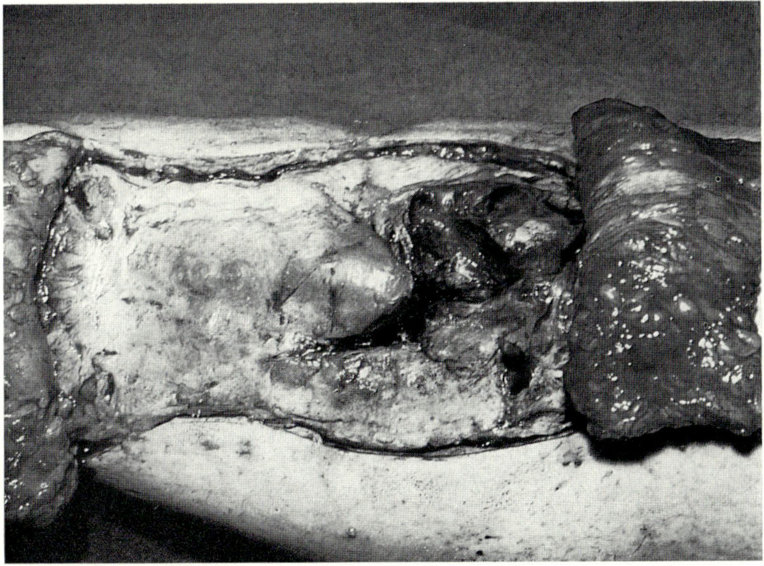

Fig. 22. Wide exposure of the bone defect. After bone grafting the excess of flap tissue with good blood supply allows closure without tension.

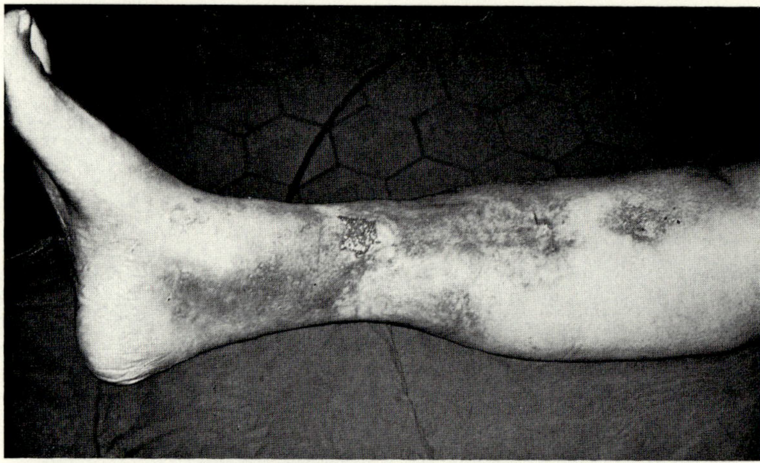

Fig. 23. Case with permanent ulcer in a circular scar after open fracture.

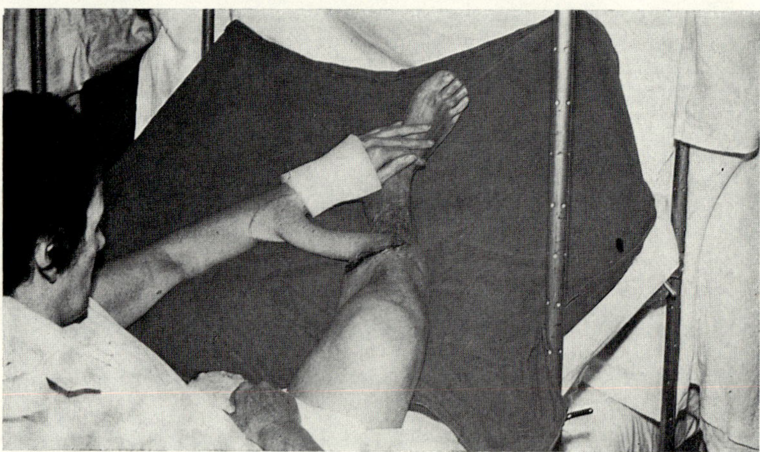

Fig. 24. We can recognise the lack of soft tissue in this picture. A tubed pedicle has been brought to the leg.

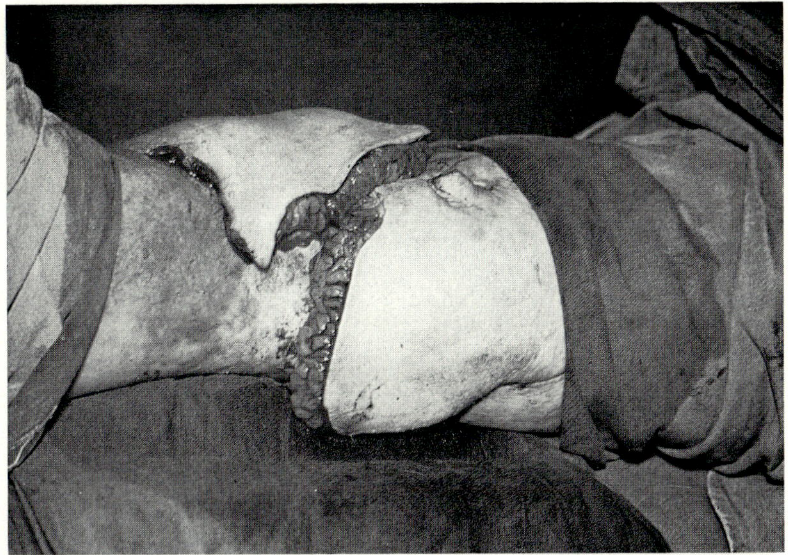

Fig. 25. The flap tissue is adapted to the defect.

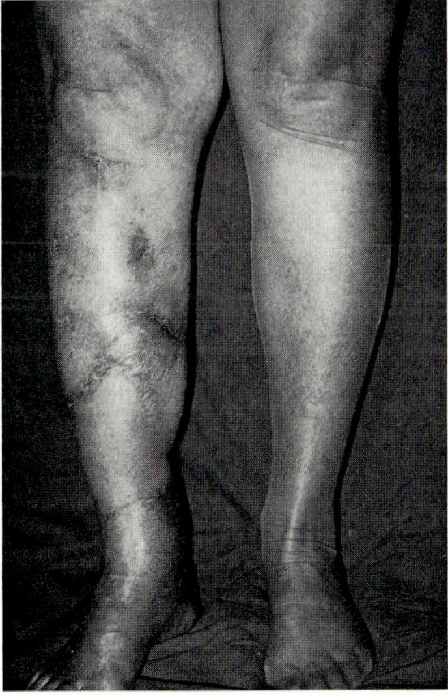

Fig. 26. Result.

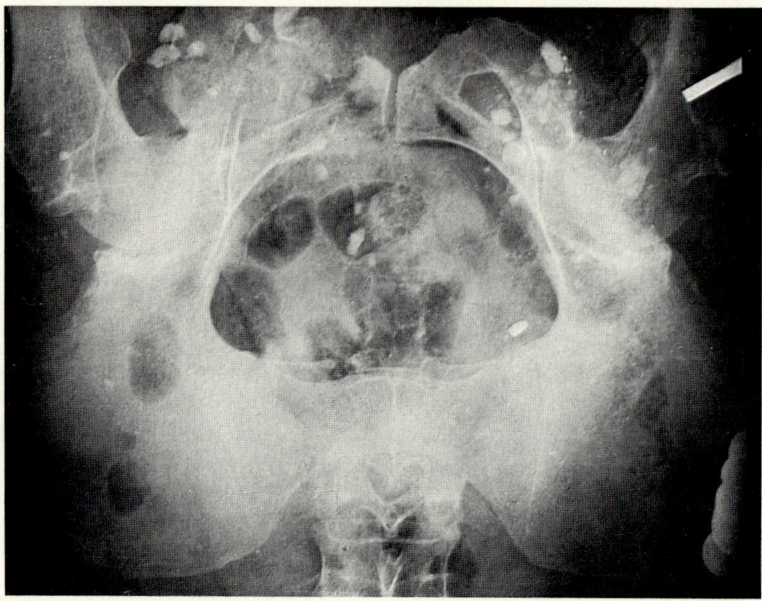

Fig. 27. A severe blast injury with open comminuted fracture of the pelvis, with injury to the rectum, the urethra and the soft tissues of the region of the symphysis.

In cases with circular skin defects of the lower limb (fig. 23) the tubed pedicled flap is the method of choice (fig. 24–26).

In a blast accident a young man had undergone extensive defects of tissue and bone in the region of the pelvis. Urethral fistulae were present (fig. 27 and 28). Local tubed pedicles were used for repair. Part of the flap was deepithelized. This part was brought subcutaneously to the symphysis to isolate the bone. Other parts of the flap were used to reconstruct the urethra (fig. 29–31).

Conclusions

Many casualities in trauma may benefit if a plastic surgery unit is attached to a clinic treating accident patients.

The main problems for the plastic and reconstructive surgeon in trauma are hand injuries, skin and soft tissue defects and especially combined defects.

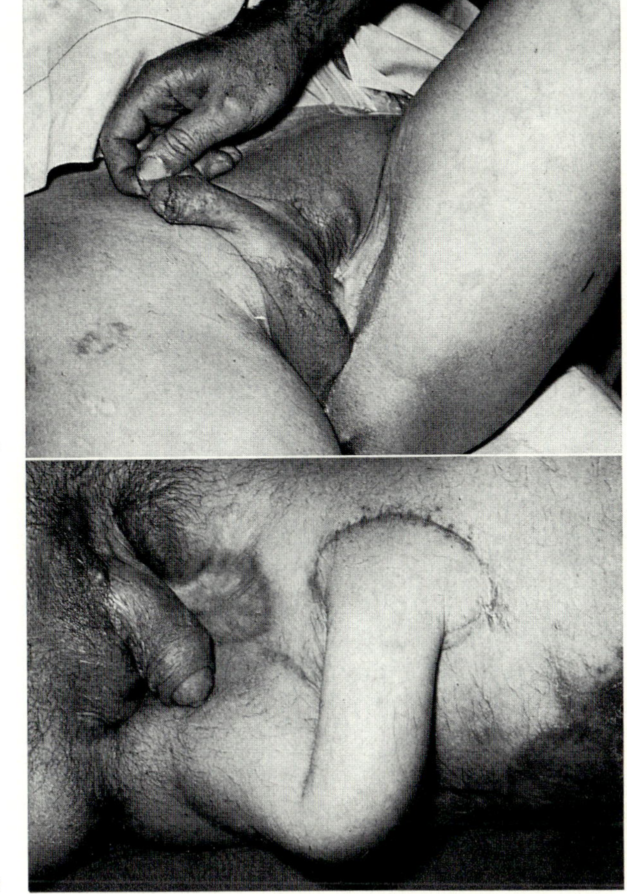

Fig. 28. After rectum amputation and wound healing several osteomyelitic and urethral fistulae are present.

Fig. 29. Nearby on the thigh a tubed pedicle is constructed and transported.

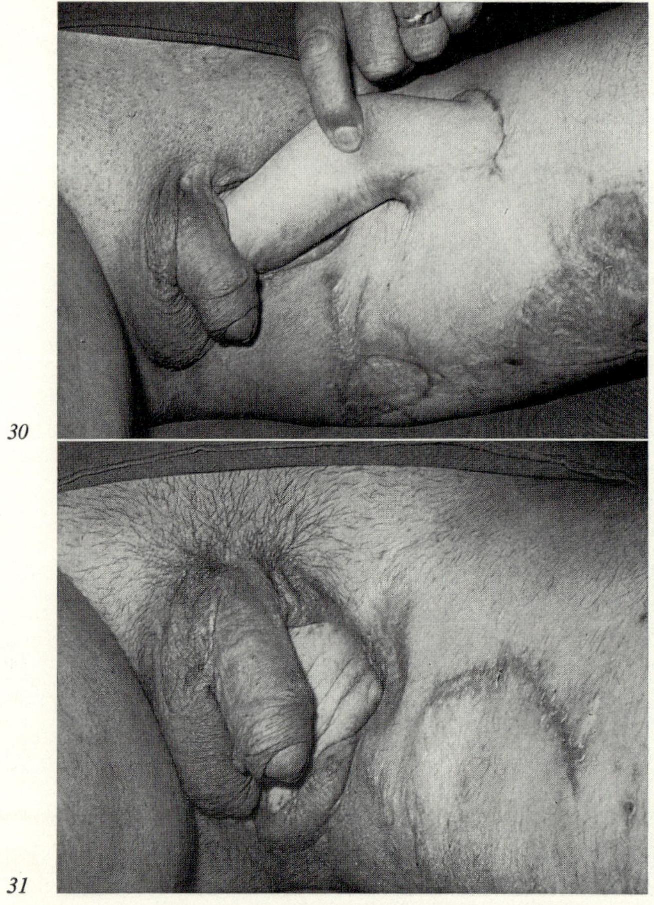

Fig. 30. The subcutaneous end of the tube is brought to the symphysis.

Fig. 31. The flap is used to close the urethral fistulae and to heal the osteo-myelitic process. As a cosmetic side-effect it imitates the lost heft part of the scrotum.

Authors' address: Dr. K. WINTSCH and Dr. E. PAMPURIK, Plastic Surgery Unit, Kantonsspital Aarau, *CH-5000 Aarau* (Switzerland)

Reconstr. Surg. Traumat., vol. 14, pp. 107–113 (Karger, Basel 1974)

Repair of Lesions
to the Flexor pollicis longus Tendon
Methods and Results

H. NIGST

Department of Surgery, Hand Surgery and Policlinic,
University of Basel, Basel

Contents

Traumatic lesions of the flexor pollicis longus tendon occur at any age, usually as cuts by glass or knives. They are therefore generally clean wounds, which may be approached primarily. It is important to assess whether one or both volar digital nerves are also severed. The restauration of sensibility should be achieved by all means in the thumb. Among our 67 cases of lesions of the flexor pollicis longus, one digital nerve was severed in 16 instances and both nerves in 4 instances. The nerves were sutured in all cases: primarily if the lesion was approached as an emergency, secondarily if a loss of sensibility was still present at the time of revision. Depending on whether magnifying spectacles or the microscope was used, two to four 6/0, 8/0 or 10/0 epineural sutures were placed.

On a follow-up of 45 patients, 34 showed no loss of sensibility, 2 displayed hyperaesthesia, while 9 had par-aesthesia in the scar or tip of the thumb.

In repairing the severed tendon of the flexor pollicis longus the method of choice appears to be the lengthening plasty, which was first described by ROUHIER [1950] and about which we have already reported earlier [NIGST and MEGEVAND, 1956 and NIGST, 1961a and b].

Provided a proper indication and good technique the lengthening plasty has proved itself satisfactory over the years. It may be used for primary repair or secondary reconstruction and has become a standard procedure of our hand team.

Our Technique of the Lengthening Plasty

General principle of the method: The distal stump of the tendon is identified, measured and resected. By means of a proximal Z plasty the remaining tendon is elongated, pulled distally and finally reinserted at the distal phalanx.

As any other delicate operative method the lengthening plasty is not always an easy procedure and should only be performed by surgeons trained in hand surgery. Unless this is the case, it is better to diagnose the lesion, close the wound and have a specialist do a secondary reconstruction.

Incision: In the case of a fresh lesion, the site of the wound (usually a transverse cut), dictates the further incision. In such cases we extend the incision on the radial midlateral side and in a semicircular curve around the thenar (fig. 1). In the case of a secondary approach we prefer to use Bruner's zigzag incision (fig. 2).

Preparation of distal stump: The severed tendon sheath is sparsely excised in order to preserve at least one, better two pulleys. The distal tendon stump is usually easy to identify, especially when the distal phalanx is flexed. Depending on the length of the distal stump, the further procedure may be planed. A distal stump of 0.5–2.5 cm generally permits a lengthening plasty of the tendon whereas 3.0 cm is considered the limit. In such extreme cases the site of the tendon muscle junction proximal to the carpal tunnel should be inspected first. If lengthening is feasible the distal stump is dissected up to its insertion in the phalanx and cut there. Care should be taken to preserve – when ever possible – part of the tendon sheath (fig. 3).

Search for the proximal end: The proximal stump of the flexor pollicis longus is often pulled back and harder to find. It may then be identified in the thenar region and should always be marked with a

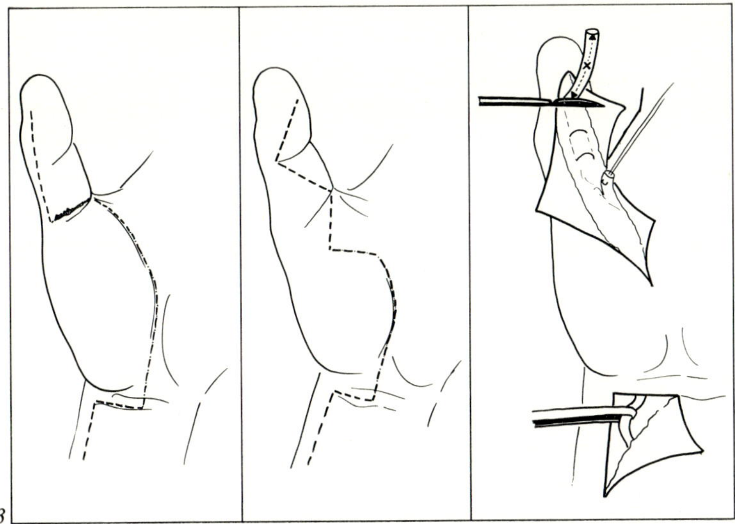

Fig. 1. Line of incision in cases of primary repair. The incision around the thenar is needed only when there are difficulties in finding the proximal tendon stump.

Fig. 2. Bruner type incision in cases of secondary repair.

Fig. 3. Dissection of the distal tendon stump. X indicates the length of elongation of the proximal stump at the wrist level.

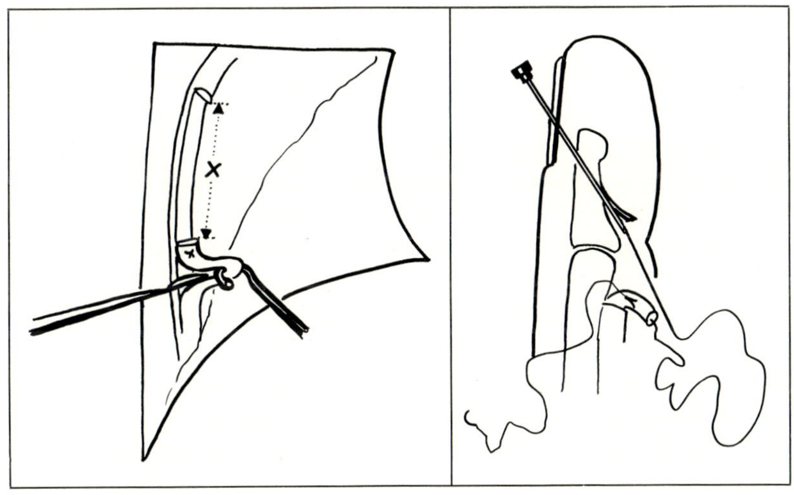

Fig. 4. Technique of elongation. One half of the tendon is cut and fixed back at a distance X distally. Thereafter the second half of the tendon is cut distally permitting a side-to-side suture of 1–2 cm.

Fig. 5. Technique of tendon insertion. A cannula is inserted through the hole made by a Kirschner wire and serves as a guide for the needle of the Lengemann suture.

thread. In secondary procedures the freeing of the tendon may be difficult due to adhesions. Careful pulling to and fro of the tendon will permit to locate the adhesions within the tendon sheath, which then are cut blindly with the scissors. If the tendon is fully pulled back to the carpus – converting it into a free graft – the holding thread should mark the route in the distal direction. In older lesions it may appear difficult to pull the club-shaped end of the cut tendon through the pulleys. In such cases either the swollen end is resected – provided enough lengthening is possible – or a wedge-like excision is performed, a method we prefer.

Lengthening of the tendon: The junction of the tendon and muscle is dissected proximal to the carpal tunnel. The Z plasty should be performed at a level proximal to the wrist so that the suture will not enter the carpal tunnel nor encroach on the median nerve when the wrist and the thumb are extended. If it does, it is advisable to split the retinaculum and leeve it open. There should be at least one, better 2 cm side-to-side contact at the suture site of the Z plasty, otherwise there would be too much weakening of the tendon. Our technique is illustrated in figure 4. The procedure is atraumatic and allows for an exact lengthening.

Tendon insertion at the phalanx: The distal insertion of the lengthened tendon is done after Bunnell's transosseous technique. A periostal flap is prepared underneath the original tendon insertion and flipped back. From there a K wire of 1–1.2 mm diameter is drilled in an oblique direction perforating the nail distally to the matrix. The K wire is replaced by a hollow cannula and the Bunnell pull-out wire or Lengemann suture holding the tendon is pulled through it (fig. 5). If too large, the rest of the original tendon is flattened and sutured to the newly inserted tendon. After release of the tourniquet and careful hemostasis a suction drainage is placed in the wound for 48 h. Finally, the thumb is immobilized in a slightly flexed position by means of a dorsal plaster splint with the wrist in a neutral position for 3 weeks, after which active exercises are started.

Indications for the lengthening plasty and its alternative: As direct flexor tendon sutures (primary and secondary) are seldom successful in the thumb, we consider a lengthening plasty to be indicated in practically all tendon transections up to the height of the metacarpophalangeal joint of the thumb. Whether or not the described technique may be used

Table I. Results of repair of flexor pollicis longus

Operative procedure	Number of cases	Total active flexion, degrees				Loss of extension
		over 60	30–60	less than 30	none	
Lengthening plasty	20	6	6	7	1	7
Free graft	11	1	5	1	4	1
Primary suture	2[1]	0	0	2	0	2
Secondary suture	4	0	1	2	1	2
Tendon transfer	4	0	2	1	1	0
Reinsertion	1	1	0	0	0	1
Tenolysis	1	0	1	0	0	0
Tenodesis	2	0	0	0	2	0
Total	45	8	15	13	9	13

1 Partially severed tendons.

depends on the distance between the transverse carpal ligament and the muscle-tendon junction. There are two alternative possibilities to choose from: a free graft of the palmaris longus or plantaris tendon and a transfer of the flexor superficialis IV tendon as described by MICHON and VILAIN [1968], which we prefer to perform in children.

Results after operative repair of the flexor pollicis longus tendon: Of the already mentioned 67 patients that had a tendon repair, 45 could be reviewed. Table I shows the distribution of the different operative methods and our preference for the lengthening plasty and the tendon grafting. Of 20 lengthening plasties, 19 displayed active flexion and only one acted as a tenodesis because of adhesions. The indicated values of active flexion take into account a possible loss of extension. This is the case mainly in the group with less than 30° of flexion and amounts on average to 20° (between 5 and 40°). In the cases treated by a free tendon graft, adhesions were observed more frequently and active flexion was on average more restricted than after lengthening plasties.

In this series, we have only 4 tendon transfers, 3 of which in children (5, 7 and 13 years old) and one in a man of 35. In the latter the flexion deficit compared with the uninjured side is only of 20°. Despite this good return of function we could not classify him in the best group as this patient had only 60° of active flexion on the uninjured side. In 3 of 4 secondary sutures active flexion could be restored. All these lesions with one exception were located in the thenar or about the carpal joint. The results of direct and primary suture of only partially cut tendons were disappointing while the cases with reinsertion displayed an active flexion of over 60°.

Discussion

The lengthening plasty of the flexor pollicis longus tendon ist a good method as a primary and secondary procedure as well. In our opinion a clean, fresh lesion of the flexor pollicis longus distal to the metacarpophalangeal joint and without major soft tissue damage should be approached primarily. In borderline cases we may consider also a free tendon graft and transfer of flexor superficialis IV, but both procedures are better done secondarily after secure wound healing. This also holds true for the tendon repair in the thenar region where a primary suture only exceptionally gives a good result.

In children we prefer the tendon transfer to the graft, because postoperative care is relatively simple and reeducation usually easy. Another indication for the tendon transfer is seen in old lesions, where the flexor muscle has lost its motor function. We have grouped our results from the surgeons standpoint by measuring the active flexion. However, for the patient some other criteria appear to be important as well. Stability of the thumb is almost as important as active movement and might be reached when flexor pollicis longus is adherent. Yet this is only acceptable if the interphalangeal joint alone is stabilised, and no passive flexion of the distal phalanx occurs during an abduction movement due to adhesions in the region of the thenar or of the wrist. One might therefore discuss primary tenodesis between the distal tendon stump and the proximal phalanx – as it is done in isolated cuts of the flexor profundus tendons of the other fingers – as an operative procedure. We have performed such a primary tenodesis of the thumb only twice in elderly patients with pre-existing limited movement of the interphalangeal joint. The good results of tendon reconstruction seem to prove that we may ask reestablishment of stability *and* flexion movement as well.

Summary

Results of treatment of 45 sections of flexor pollicis longus tendon are given. For lesions with a distal stump less than 3 cm lengthening and insertion of the proximal stump is a good method of treatment. When the distal stump is longer a free graft or transfer of flexor superficialis from the ring finger is advocated. The technique of tendon elongation and insertion is described in details.

References

BUNNELL, St.: Surgery of the hand (Lippincott, Philadelphia 1956).

MICHON, J. et VILAIN, R.: Lésions traumatiques des tendons de la main (Masson, Paris 1968).

NIGST, H. et MEGEVAND, R. P.: La réparation du long fléchisseur propre du pouce. Technique de l'élongation du tendon. Helv. chir. Acta 23: 456 (1956).

NIGST, H.: Zur Frage der primären Versorgung der Beugesehnenverletzung im Niemandsland der Hand. Msch. Unfallheilk. 2: 63 (1961a).

NIGST, H.: Ergebnisse der Sehnenplastiken der Hand. Arch. klin. Chir. 299 (1961b).

ROUHIER, G.: La restauration du tendon long fléchisseur du pouce sans sacrifice du tendon primitif. J. Chir., Paris 66: 8 (1950).

Author's address: Prof. Dr. H. NIGST, Department of Surgery, University of Basel, Hand Surgery and Policlinic, *CH-4000 Basel* (Switzerland)

Reconstr. Surg. Traumat., vol. 14, pp. 114–135 (Karger, Basel 1974)

Vascular and Nervous Complications in Injuries of the Knee Joint

C. E. Ottolenghi[1] and C. H. Traversa

Department of Orthopaedic Surgery and Traumatology,
Italian Hospital, Buenos Aires

Contents

Severe injuries to the knee joint were observed in 1,375 cases in the last years. From this total amount it appears that despite the apparent vulnerability of the vasculo-nervous elements that run through the knee joint, injuries of these structures are relatively rare. According to our statistics, 44 cases (3.2 %) were found. This figure is near to that reported by other authors. Injuries in which vascular and nervous complications were observed are described in table I.

---

1   Consulting Professor, Faculty of Medicine, University of Buenos Aires.

Table I. Vascular and nervous complications; 821 cases (meniscus excluded)

Traumatism	Cases	Vascular injuries	Nervous injuries	Vasculo-nervous injuries
Fracture lower end of femur	203	6	1	–
Fracture tibial plateau and upper third of tibia	387	10	4	5
Ligamentous injury and Harry Platt's Syndrome	205	–	11	–
Dislocation of knee joint	23	3	1	–
Severe bruise of knee joint	2	2	–	–
Open fracture produced by weapon	1	–	1	–
Total	821	21	18	5

Most of these injuries were suffered by men; there were 38 males (1 bilateral), and 5 females.

The ages were as follows:

Age, years	Cases
10–19	5
20–29	13
30–39	9
40–49	6
50–59	5
60–69	5

It appears that these injuries are mostly observed in middle-aged patients. No cases under 10 nor over 70 years of age were seen.

They were produced by the following accidents:

Etiology	Cases
Traffic	28
Work	6
Home	2
Sport	5
Shotgun wound	1
Explosion	1

21 of the total amount of vasculo-nervous injuries were of vascular origin and 18 of nervous nature; in 5 cases, combined vascular and nerve injuries were observed.

Vascular Injuries (26 cases, 1.89 %)

Although the vascular component is constant in every traumatism and especially in fractures, injuries to the great vessels in civilian life are infrequent.

Fineschi [1958, 1959] presented 58 cases of which 17 were at the level of the knee joint.

De Bakey and Simeone [1946] observed 2 % of vascular complications, the same rate as given by Chippault over a total of 40,000 traumatisms. In 92 of 296 cases, they observed that the popliteal artery was damaged; in 8 cases the tibio-fibular trunk, in 22 the posterior tibial artery, and in 16 the anterior tibial artery.

Lena and d'Allaines observed that in 22.9 % of their cases the popliteal artery was affected.

The popliteal artery with its branches, the tibio-fibular and anterior tibial trunks may be damaged due to the traumatic lesions mentioned before.

Theoretically, the popliteal artery injuries should not be serious as far as the peripheral blood irrigation of the limb is concerned, because the collateral branches of this artery that surround the knee could maintain the distal blood flow in the case of damage to the principal trunk, but in the practice, the popliteal artery injury provokes ischemic lesions of the limb beneath the site of traumatism.

Our statistics confirm this, as 11 of 24 cases had to be amputated; the Volkmann syndrome was present in 12 and only 3 recovered. Vascular injuries may be caused by direct or indirect mechanism or both at a time. In fractures, a bony fragment can produce a direct bruise of the arterial trunk. The displaced segment in anterior or posterior dislocations is often the compression factor and consequently the cause of arterial damage. In cases of fracture, the indirect compression due to tension hematoma in the fibular groove is added to the direct traumatism.

Very important anatomical structures that must be taken into account – especially pointed out by Lena and d'Allaines – are the elements that the popliteal artery crosses at the level of the popliteal groove.

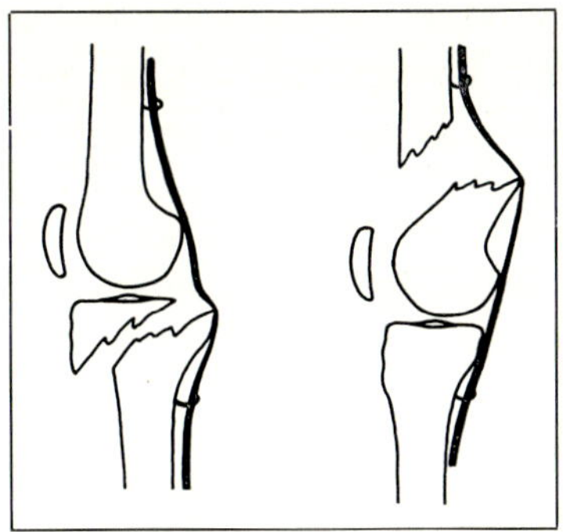

Fig. 1. The popliteal artery may be damaged in fractures of the lower end of the femur or upper end of the tibia. The artery runs from the anulus of the third adductor muscle to the anulus of the soleus muscle.

The popliteal artery, placed behind the bony elements of the knee, runs from the internal to the posterior aspect of the thigh at the level of the annulus of the third adductor, leaving the popliteal groove through the soleus annulus. The popliteal artery and vein meet at their upper and lower ends and are surrounded by two fibrous annuli.

If elongation of a vessel is produced by an accident, the stiffness of the aforementioned annulus does not allow the displacement of the vessels which remain elongated as a taut cord. The vessels then rupture, either by direct contusion or lack of strength (fig. 1).

Injuries to the popliteal artery have been observed in the following cases:

1. Lower Third and Supra- or Intercondylar Fractures of Femur

Of 203 cases, 7 (3.44 %) vascular complications were observed. In one case, external sciatic popliteal nerve paralysis existed. Two of these patients had an acute ischemic syndrome and were amputated. The remaining 5 presented Volkmann's ischemic syndrome (fig. 2). One of them was seen 48 h after the accident; 2 after 6 h, one after 12 h and the last one 24 months later. This indicates that despite the frequency of fractures at the lower end of the femur and the nearness of the vessels to the bone at the level of the third adductor annulus, vascular injuries, especially those producing the acute ischemic syndrome, are not very frequent.

Delayed ischemias due to exuberant fracture callus at the level of the referred annulus have been observed. Lavigne as well as Böhler consider this complication as exceptional. Scuderi and Hippolito observed only one case in 21 years. Lena and d'Allaines reported 11 cases and Seni reported 3. Cauchoix and Deburge [1969] did not see any of these complications. The injury is produced by direct contusion of the lower fragment which is displaced backwards.

2. Fractures of the Upper End of the Tibia

Of 379 cases, 14 (3.71 %) presented vascular complications. These fractures are of bad prognosis as far as vascular complications are concerned. Jourdan [1959] calls them 'fractures with gangrene'. This author presents 7 personal cases of 149 registered. Ellis reported that amputations had to be performed in 5 cases out of 225, although radiographically the injuries did not appear to be serious.

Merle d'Aubigné *et al.* [1959] calls attention to the fact that delayed vascular disturbances appear in apparently unimportant injuries.

The most frequent type of fracture that may give rise to ischemic syndrome is that of the tibial plateau presenting an oblique fracture line upwards and backwards that begins immediately below the anterior tibial tuberosity and passes near to the articular border (fig. 3). In certain cases the displacement and dislocation of the fragments are not very important (fig. 4). In the great majority of cases there is more than one fracture line, especially at the level of the external tibial plateau which is strongly displaced outwards and may produce either external sciatic popliteal nerve paralysis (fig. 5) or injury to the anterior tibial artery. The popliteal artery is the more affected vessel; the tibio-peroneal trunk or the anterior or posterior tibial arteries are less often injured. Fortunately, not all cases of important displacements described provoke ischemic complications, and these may also be observed in cases not suspected radiographically.

It is therefore very important to find out at a patient's clinical examination whether there is any peripheral circulatory disturbance. In 7 subjects there was acute ischemic syndrome; one patient arrived 24 h after the accident, 2 arrived after 48 h, another one after 6 days, and one a month later. The popliteal artery was injured in 5 cases; the tibio-peroneal trunk in 2.

The syndrome was delayed in 7 patients, who were followed up

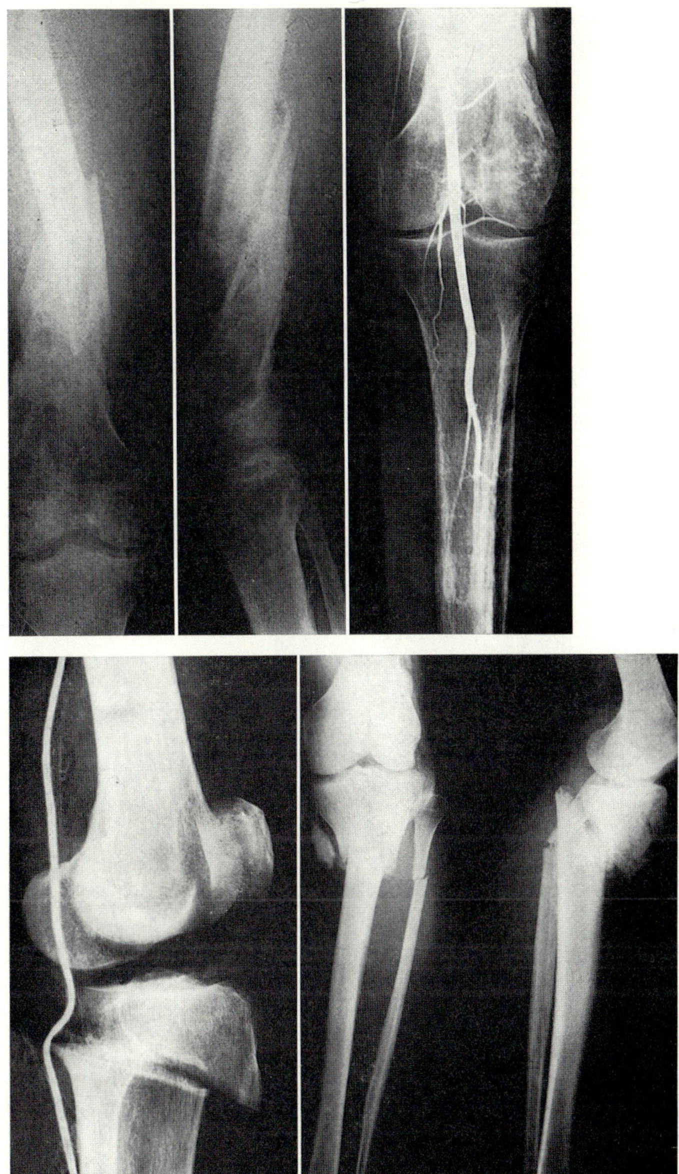

Fig. 2. Fracture of the lower third of the femur. Arteriography. Volkmann's syndrome.

Fig. 3. Oblique fracture directed forwards and backwards. The fracture focus and its connection with the popliteal artery.

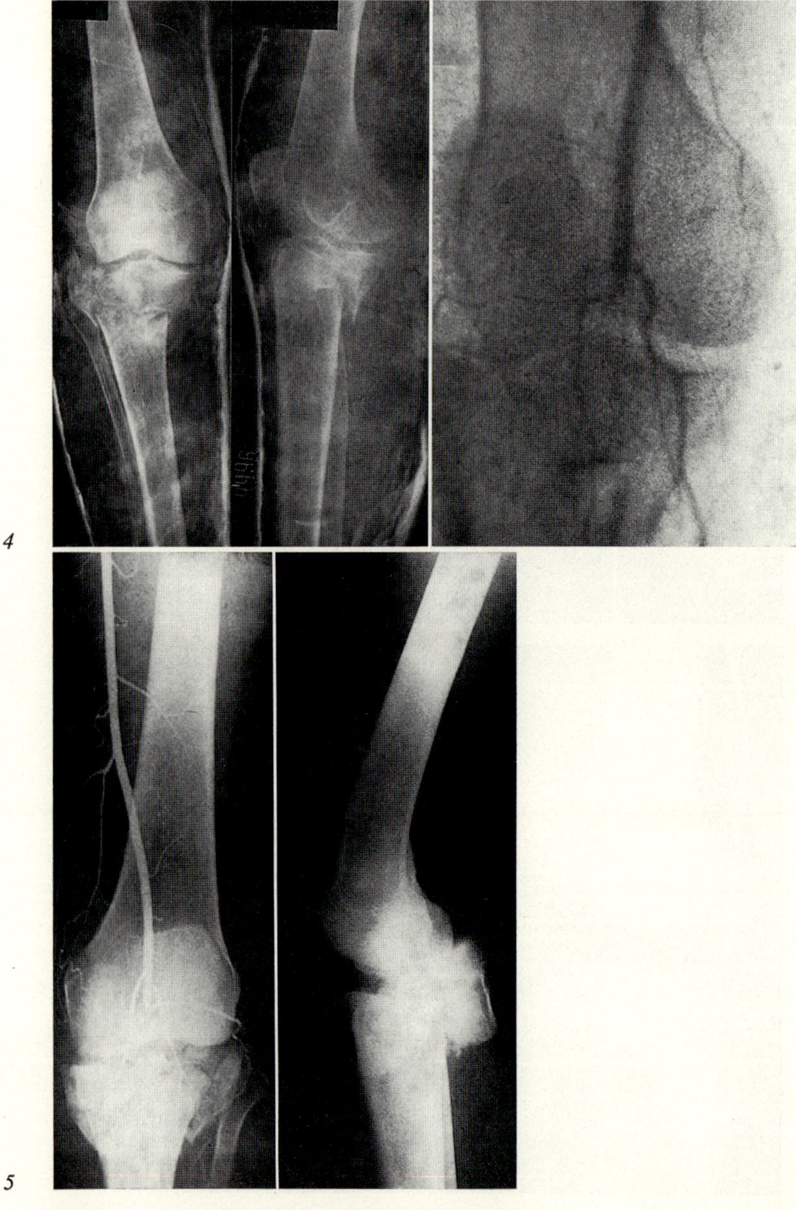

Fig. 4. Comminuted tibial plateau fracture without great displacement. Acute ischemic syndrome. Arteriography. Gangrene.

Fig. 5. Tibial plateau and upper end fibular fracture. Great displacement. Acute ischemic syndrome. Arteriography. Gangrene.

between 36 h and 7 years. In 5 cases an important displacement of the fragments was seen, but in 2 of them it was minimum.

In 5 cases the popliteal artery and in 2 the tibio-peroneal trunk were damaged. In one of the acute cases there was also an external sciatic popliteal nerve paralysis, whilst in the chronic cases, two of them presented the same injury and in another one, both the external and internal sciatic popliteal nerves were injured.

Dislocations

This injury is observed after severe traumatisms. Dislocation may be either anterior or posterior (fig. 6). We observed 23 cases of dislocation of the knee joint, in 3 of which the popliteal artery was damaged, 2 patients had to be amputated and the remainder recovered completely. The rate of vascular injuries varies according to the different authors. KENNEDY observed vascular disturbances in 56 % of 25 dislocations. CALLAHAN [1962] reported only 3 complications in 20 cases. HOOVER [1961] reported 14 cases and 9 ischemic syndromes. It is argued which of each type of dislocation is most severe. KENNEDY supports that the anterior, whilst CALLAHAN [1962] believes that the posterior dislocation is more serious. Dislocations produced in anatomical sections showed us that in forward displacements, the artery is introduced into the intercondylar incisure and can be freed; whilst in the posterior dislocation, the impact is direct from the tibial plateau.

Closed Injuries without Bony Lesion

In certain cases the vascular damage is produced without affecting the skeleton as in the following observation:

Case 11: Work accident. His right leg was caught in a pulley which rose and threw him a certain distance. The patient was hospitalized with an acute ischemic syndrome.

Case 9: Contusion of the popliteal groove by work accident (the patient was compressed between two tramways). He arrived after the accident. Enlargement of the artery was found. It was opened and coagulums removed. The artery was sutured previous to heparin injection. The patient recovered (fig. 7).

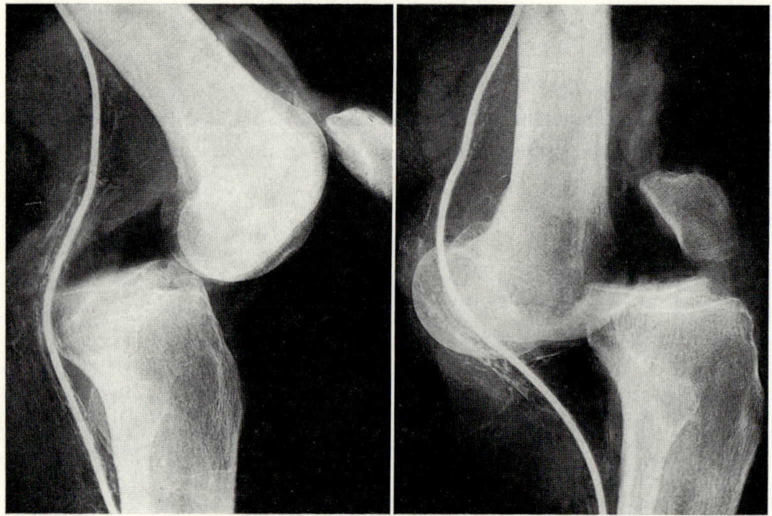

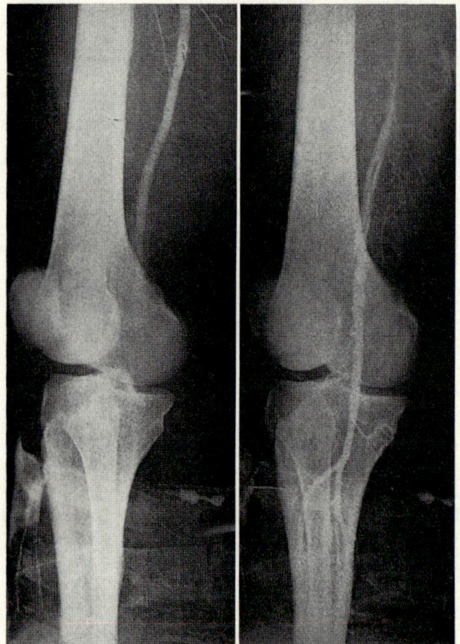

Fig. 6. The popliteal artery in anterior and posterior dislocations.

Fig. 7. Closed injury. Section of the popliteal artery. Patient 62 years old. Operated on 6 h after the accident. Suture of the artery. Recovery.

Symptomatology

Acute ischemia. The 4 Ps syndrome described by GRIFFITHS and LIPSCOMB can be applied here: pain, pallor, pulseness and paralysis. The most important signs are:

Pain: Different from that produced by the trauma. It does not disappear with rest, immobilization or analgesics; it is persistent and increasing. The localization is distant from the osteoarticular injury.

Pallor: The skin is livid presenting sometimes areas of coloration. The fingers appear cyanotic.

Paralysis: Generally the paresis is noticeable below the level of the injury of the limb, but total paralysis is less frequent. It appears rapidly accompanied by sensitive disorders which are not sistematized as hypoesthetic or anesthetic types.

Pulseness: This is a sign of great importance and must often be taken. In some cases the pedial and posterior tibial pulses may be conserved even in great vascular injuries, because the blood may flow in the adventitia or intima during the first hours after the accident, but later on it decreases till disappearing. In spasms or compressions the blood flow may reappear after the treatment or turn out to be a simple transitory modification.

Temperature: Coldness is an evident sign of peripheral collapse or shock.

Muscular retraction: This appears a few hours after the traumatism and is a sign of arterial injury. The posterior compartment is especially affected, producing muscular rigidity as seen in tetanic lesions; this sign is characteristic of injury to the anterior tibial artery.

Peripheral vascular disturbances: Disappearance of cutaneous veins, decrease of capillary return circulation and slight edema are present.

Oscillometry. It is important to assess arterial blood flow and its periodical control at different levels of the limb. Oscillometry is as valuable as arteriography in the diagnosis of vascular injury.

In the *subacute ischemic syndrome,* pain is less intense though it does not disappear with rest. There are changes in the distal local temperature and coloration of the limb, but no coldness or pallor to the degree observed in total occlusions.

The pedial and posterior tibial pulses may be perceivable but to a smaller extent than on the opposite side. The sign of return venous repletion is present in most of the cases and there is no paralysis. Oscillometry is easier to perform than in the complete acute syndrome and oscillations of lesser extent than in normal cases may be found. Repeated oscillometry may be useful. In these cases as well as in the acute ones arteriography is effective.

Arteriography. It is very important to localize the place of the obstruction and demonstrate if there is collateral blood flow. Despite the fact that some authors consider it useless or dangerous, we believe that in all cases of acute ischemia, arteriography is a valuable resource. It is not essential in cases presenting irreversible gangrene phenomena which are seen too late and also not in those in whom the symptoms are so clear that surgical exploration is mandatory.

Arteriography may demonstrate a filiform image as seen in spasms, the obstruction may be either lineal as in ruptures or cupule-shaped as in thrombosis. The lesions of the intima may demonstrate in the first hours an irregular tracing at the level of the injury; the ruptures may also show shadows as observed in vascular hematomas. Arterio-venous aneurysms can also be visualized. The use of vasodilator solutions (20 ml of sulution at 20 %) is recommended.

FORSTER *et al.* [1963] and LUMKIN *et al.* [1958] are in favor of this procedure. SPENCER [1962] advises it in all suspected fractures or traumas with large hematomas and edemas in which the clinical observation cannot be cleared up. It can be argued that this method does not demonstrate the exact nature of the injury; i. e. whether the arrest is due to anatomical lesion, spasm or hematoma. Notwithstanding, arteriography is an important complementary method in knee joint injuries and should be performed in the proper cases.

Evolution – Prognosis

It is necessary to emphasize the imperious need to find out the clinical signs of ischemia immediately after the accident. In every knee fracture or dislocation, the physicians who first take care of the patient should be aware that a peripheral circulatory disturbance might be present and be able to apply the corresponding urgent measures.

The muscles do not tolerate an ischemia exceeding 8–12 h. After this limit of time degenerative phenomena become irreversible, although blood flow may be restored subsequently.

According to the foregoing the diagnosis and therapeutical measures should be applied within that period. Every well-organized hospital for the care of injured should rely on trained surgeons who are able to perform arteriographies and vascular sutures. The most convenient in these cases is the close collaboration between the Orthopedic and Cardio-Vascular Departments. If the patient has been primarily treated in a hospital lacking this equipment, he should be immediately transferred to a better equipped center.

The evolution and prognosis depend upon the arterial damage suffered, the earliness of the diagnosis and quality of treatment applied.

The artery may present functional or organic damages: (1) functional – spasm; (2) organic – compression (intimal injury), contusion (intimal and middle layer injury), elongation (incomplete or complete anatomical section).

Vascular spasm is a constant reaction in every direct or indirect arterial trauma. The pure vascular spasm without injury to the walls of the vessel is very difficult to find. LENA and D'ALLAINES, among others, have demonstrated that in practice vascular spasms without apparent external injury present more or less important intimal lesions that partially limit the blood flow in the first moments, but this is rapidly stopped by the thrombosis which finally obstructs completely the light of the vessel.

The pure spasm may provoke a transitory ischemic syndrome, clinically externalized by either immediate total recovery or delayed ischemic syndrome.

Regarding the circulatory interruption due to arterial injury or section, the local clinical conditions will vary, because in the first case the ischemic phenomena are pure, whilst in the second case an increasingly progressive hematoma distending the tissues and provoking signs of acute anemia is added.

The prognosis of popliteal artery injuries is bad. HOOVER reported that amputation was necessary in more than 50 % of the cases. Of 34 patients, he obtained excellent results in 10, fair results in 6, and 18 were amputated. LENA and D'ALLAINES had 10 excellent results, 8 fair results and 36 amputations (66.66 %) in 54 cases.

The prognosis depends fundamentally on the time elapsed since the accident. According to the authors mentioned last, in the first 10 h only 11 % of the cases had to be amputated.

In our statistics of 25 cases, 11 were amputated, 7 complained of fracture of the upper third of the tibia, 2 dislocation of the knee, 2 fractures of the lower end of the femur.

The time of evolution was as follows:

Time	Cases
24 h	3
48 h	2
72 h	3
6 days	1 (bilateral)
1 month	1

Two cases had an excellent evolution; both were treated within the first 6 h of the accident. First case: closed traumatism without fracture; ischemic syndrome with large tension hematoma; section of the popliteal artery and vein; suture; recovery 100 %. Second case: posterior dislocation of the knee joint; exploration; the patient was hospitalized on the same day; his infrapatellar wound was treated and the dislocation reduced; no pulse was found and immediate surgery was performed.

Fair Results

A case of closed traumatism with ischemic syndrome. Exploration. Injury of intima on the site of bifurcation of the popliteal artery. Suture. Partial ischemic signs: loss of first and fifth toes. Limb conserved.

Volkmann's Syndrome (12 cases)

Fracture upper end of tibia: 7 cases; fracture lower end of femur: 5 cases.

Four recent cases: 1 fracture tibial plateau: seen at 36 h; 1 fracture lower end femur: seen at 48 h; 1 fracture tibial plateau: seen at 48 h, and 1 fracture tibial platea: seen at 72 h.

The remaining 8 were observed between 50 days and 7 years.

In the first three cases observed between 36 and 48 h after the accident the ischemic syndrome was stopped. In the fourth case the acute syndrome was severe and the vascular bundle was surgically explored. The patient conserved the limb although he presented the Volkmann syndrome.

Time	Cases	Site of injury
50 days	1	tibia
60 days	2	1 tibia and 1 femur
6 months	2	femur
1 year	1	femur
1½ years	1	tibia
7 years	1	tibia

The individual interruption of the anterior and posterior tibial arteries generally does not produce serious residual lesions for the compensatory anastomosis, but the high injury of the trunks, especially that of the anterior tibial artery, may give rise to an acute necrotic syndrome of the muscles of the antero-external region of the leg. Intense pain and permanent muscular contracture at this level are present.

The sole popliteal vein injury is rare; locally a tension hematoma is produced but generally the superficial blood flow is maintained. However, cases of venous gangrene have been described; the symptomatology appears more lately than in arterial injuries, between the 4th and 8th days. The predominant signs besides the aforementioned are edema and progressive cyanosis.

Once more we insist upon the importance of early diagnosis. Unfortunately, when the acute occlusion syndrome persists for more than 12 h, prognosis is very serious.

The patient's age and the possibile preexistance of known or unknown arteriopathies are an aggravating factor in the prognosis of popliteal artery injury. However, one of our excellent cases who totally recovered, after arterial and vein suture, was 62 years old.

Treatment

Acute vascular complications have to be managed with the greatest urgency. Different circumstances have to be differentiated.

1. Injury presenting vascular disturbance from the beginning. (a) Reduction of the bony injury under anesthesia as soon as possible. (b) If the ischemic signs do not disappear after removing the eventual compressive element: arteriography. (c) Surgical exploration of the focus.

Examination of the artery and vein. The artery may present spasm, bruise or longitudinal section: (1) if spasm without pulse was observed at the distal fragment, lukewarm compresses would be placed; if the pulse does not appear (which happens more frequently), arteriectomy, removal of the blood clot, and examination of the intima; if, as often observed, endo-arterial injury exists, arteriectomy of the affected segment and suture of its both ends, if the separation is less than 4 cm; (2) in evident contusion of the arterial walls – arteriectomy and the same behavior as in former case. (3) longitudinal section – if no intimal injury exists, transversal sutture to avoid stretching of the vessel; (4) arterial section – generally the ends are retracted; if they cannot be approached, internal saphenous venous graft to maintain the continuity of the vessel; (5) in injuries of the popliteal artery the repair with foreign materials (teflon, dacron, etc.) have failed as far as we know.

We are not going to describe the technique of arterial or venous sutures. No hemostatic tourniquet should be applied in reconstructive or exploratory vascular surgery. Complementary treatment with vasodilators and anticoagulants are of help but the fundamental treatment is to restore the continuity of the vessel as rapidly as possible. The operation should be finished with a wide superficial and deep aponeurectomy until opening the soleus annulus, as advised by MERLE D'AUBIGNÉ, to avoid post-operatory edemas, that favor delayed blood flow, thrombosis, etc.; postoperatory compressive plaster casts should be avoided. Stable osteosynthesis or skeletal tractions are advised to maintain reductions.

2. Injuries that may give rise to vascular disturbances. These must be early managed to avoid subacute or delayed ischemic phenomena that may produce the Volkmann syndrome.

3. In cases with ischemia already established the reconstructive and conservative management is ineffective. Unfortunately, in evident massive ischemic signs it is useless to make oscillometries or arteriographies. These patients have to be amputated at the site of the vascular injury.

Nerve Injuries

Of the total figure mentioned above, 23 knee traumatisms (1.6 %) nerve injuries were observed.

These nerve injuries were seen in the following cases:

Injury	Cases
Ligamentous injuries: Harry Platt's syndrome	11
Fracture of upper end of tibia and fibula	9
Fracture of lower end of femur	1
Dislocation of knee joint	1
Section for shotgun wound	1

23 cases of the total presented external sciatic popliteal nerve paralysis, in 3 of them internal sciatic popliteal nerve paralysis was added and in 5 there was a combined vasculo-nervous injury. In 4 of these cases the external sciatic popliteal nerve was damaged and in one both nerves were injured. There were 20 males and 3 females.

Etiology	Cases
Traffic accident	14
Work accident	4
Sport accident	3
Shotgun wound	1

Nerve injuries associated with knee traumatism generally occur in accidents that affect the capsulo-ligamentous complex. Of 23 of our cases, 11 patients (50 %) presented the syndrome described by PLATT [1940]. In these cases the mechanism of the nerve injury was both indirect – because the traumatism did not take place at the level of the injured point – and direct – by elongation of the external sciatic popliteal nerve over the bony structures with which it is related (fig. 8). In 8 cases the paralysis was associated with fracture of the tibial plateau. In these cases the trauma may act directly on the nerve trunk. Only in one case of fracture of the lower end of the femur, external sciatic popliteal nerve paralysis was observed, and in one case the injury was produced by a shotgun that affected the external aspect of the knee. Isolated internal sciatic popliteal nerve paralysis was not observed in any of our cases.

The internal and external sciatic popliteal nerves run across the knee. Both nerves arise from the major sciatic nerve which is generally divided into two branches at the level of the popliteal rhombus. The first branch, the larger one, descends vertically and introduces itself into the soleus

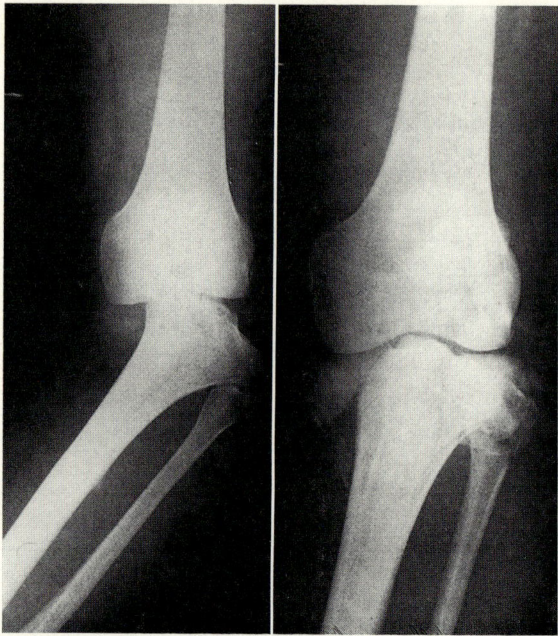

Fig. 8. Paralysis of the external sciatic popliteal nerve. Varus deviation.

annulus placed behind the popliteal vessels. The other branch runs obliquely downwards and outwards following the internal border of the bicipital tendon and laying completely superficially underneath the aponeurosis. On descending it crosses by the external femoral condyle and the insertion of the external gemellus muscle, placed behind the fibular head and, surrounding the neck of this bone, passes between it and the lateral peroneus longus, dividing finally into two branches: the tibialis anterior and the cutaneous muscles. The rupture of the collateral ligaments, especially the external ones, sometimes combined with injuries to the cruciate ligaments gives rise to the damage of the external sciatic popliteal nerve. The association of fibular head fracture with external collateral ligament tear that provokes paralysis of the satellite nerve is known as Harry Platt's syndrome. On the one hand the elongation and on the other the compression or tear give rise to irreversible paralysis due to the lability of the nerve.

Less frequently, injuries to both nerves of the leg (internal and external sciatic popliteal nerves) are observed. When this takes place the injury sets up at the level of the major sciatic nerve. In most of the cases the damages are of the dissociated type with persistence of external sciatic popliteal nerve deficit. Because of the accident, a severe varus deviation with or without knee dislocation is produced.

The symptomatology is classical. The flaccid paralysis in these cases is total, comprising all the muscles inervated by the affected nerve. Sensitiveness may be totally or partially abolished. The picture is completed with lack of tendinous reflexes and tropic troubles with degenerative reactions. The partial lesion appears as a paresis which affects the corresponding muscles with sensitive troubles that may vary between hypoesthesia and hyperesthesia; tendinous reflexes may also be affected and trophic disturbances may or may not be present. Dissociative paralysis generally ends in a definitive syndrome.

From the diagnostic point of view, apart from clinical and neurological routine examinations, electrodiagnosis and electromyography are of use to determine the degree of nerve integrity: (1) deficit syndrome; (2) interruption syndrome, and (3) dissociation syndrome.

According to SEDDON [1966] the nerve injuries can be classified as: neuroapraxia (irritative syndrome); axonomesis (compressive syndrome), and neurotmesis (interruption syndrome).

Prognosis: The first and second syndromes are of good prognosis as far as functional recovery is concerned. The functional prognosis of external sciatic popliteal nerve injuries of the knee is serious. Paralysis was irreversible (neurotmesis) in 18 of 23 cases. Only 4 cases recovered: dislocation of the knee, 1; fracture of tibial plates, 1; Harry Platt's syndrome, 2. One case had to be amputated because of associated vascular injury.

Generally, the primary injury gives rise to an irreversible nerve damage because, due to the violent accident, it is roughly elongated. This has been proved in cases of late exploration in which the external sciatic popliteal nerve was found without apparent solution of continuity, but narrowed and fibrous in a noticeable area. Complete nerve section has not been observed in cases of closed injury.

Treatment

The management of nerve damages of the knee, especially of the external sciatic popliteal nerve, depends upon the type of injury: fracture or ligamentous tear.

The therapeutical behavior in ligamentous injuries should be undoubtedly the surgical reconstruction of all damaged structures. The operation must be performed within the first days after the accident. The sequelae in these cases are always due to misdiagnosis or to an incomplete primary examination.

If at exploring the ligamentous injuries, nerve paralysis were found, the damaged nerves should be explored and freed in the eventual case of compression, but generally in primary surgical exploration only neurolysis is performed.

Resection of the bruised nerve segment and neurorraphy do not give satisfactory results and the patient remains irreversibly paralyzed.

Concerning the solution of residual paralysis, we think it is an argument that should not be discussed here; the orthopedic and surgical management of sequelae of nerve injuries is a separated chapter of reconstructive surgery of the foot.

Summary

Over a total of 1,375 severe injuries of the knee joint, 45 cases (3.2 %) of vasculo-nervous complications were observed. Vascular complications were seen in 24 cases and nervous complications in 22; in 4 instances the injuries were combined.

Lesions of the popliteal artery or its branches are serious; over the total amount already mentioned, it was necessary to amputate in 11 cases; 12 patients presented the Volkmann syndrome.

In cases of fractures of the lower end of femur, upper end of tibia and knee dislocations, the importance of early diagnosis of the acute ischemic syndrome is emphasized.

Tibial plateau injuries produce the largest amount of vascular complications; urgent therapeutic behavior is indicated.

Nerve injuries were observed in 22 cases, the external sciatic popliteal nerve being almost constantly damaged. In 4 cases a combined vasculo-nervous injury was seen and in 2 paralysis of the internal sciatic popliteal nerve was added.

Prognosis of injuries to the external sciatic popliteal nerve is serious because over the total amount, in 17 cases (81 %) paralysis war irreversible.

References

ARNULF (Bureau du colombier): Documents cliniques et expérimentaux sur la contusion artérielle et leurs déductions thérapeutiques. Lyon chir. *47:* 566 (1952).

Bureau du colombier: Contribution à l'étude de la contusion artérielle; thèse, Lyon (1951).

CAHUZAC, M. et JUNG, F.: Contusion de l'artère fémorale, spasme vasculaire, syndrome de Volkmann. Rev. Orthop. *32:* 241 (1946).

CALLAHAN, J. J.: Vascular complications of the dislocation of the shoulder and knee. Clin. Congr. Vascular Complications of Skeletal Traumas (Amer. College of Surgeons, Chicago 1962).

Campbell's operative orthopaedics: vol. I, p. 60 (1963).

CARABALONA *et al.:* Ischémie aiguë du membre inférieur par traumatismes fermés du genou. Mém. Acad. Chir. *88:* 86 (1962).

COLLINS, H. A. et JACOBS, J. K.: Acute arterial injuries due to blunt trauma. J. Bone Jt Surg. *43A:* 193 (1961).

CAUCHOIX, J. and DEBURGE, A.: Recent fractures of the lower end of the femur. Reconstr. Surg. Traumat. *11:* 183 (1969).

CRAWFORD, E. S. and DE BAKEY, M. E.: The retrograde flush procedure in embolectomy and thrombectomy. Surgery *40:* 737 (1956).

CRELLIN, R. Q. and TSAPOGAS, M. J. C.: Traumatic aneurysm of the anterior tibial artery. Report of a case. J. Bone Jt Surg. *45B:* 142 (1963).

DE BAKEY, M. E. and SIMEONE, F. A.: Battle injuries of the arteries in World War II. Analysis of 2,471 cases. Ann. Surg. *123:* 534 (1946).

DE MOURGUES-CHAIX, D.: Traitement des factures des plateaux tibiaux. Rev. Chir. orthop. répar. Appar. moteur *50:* 103 (1964).

FINESCHI, G.: La cura chirurgica della sindrome de contrattura di Volkmann dell'artro inferiore. 43rd Congr. Soc. Ital. Ortop. Traumat., p. 471 (1958).

FINESCHI, G.: Le lesioni vascolari e nervose in rapporto con i traumi legati alla vita moderna. Nuovi aspetti dei traumatismi dell'apparato locomotore in rapporto con i tempi moderni. III. Relaz. al Congr. Soc. Ital. Ortop. Traumat., Roma (1959).

FISHER, G. W.: Acute arterial injuries treated by the United States Army Medical Service in Vietnam, 1965–1966. J. Trauma *7:* 844 (1967).

FONTAINE, R. et BRANZEN, P.: Un nouveau cas d'enclavement irréductible de l'artère humérale dans un foyer de fracture suscondylienne de l'humérus. Rev. Chirurg. *75:* 145 (1937).

FONTAINE, R.; WINISDOERFER, B. et MARTIN, P.: Strasbourg méd. *6:* 642 (1955).

FORSTER, E.; MOLE, L.; KUNLIN, A. et SCHOEBELEN, R.: Lésions artérielles au cours des traumatismes fermés des membres. Neuf observations personnelles. Mém. Acad. Chir. *89:* 5 (1963).

FRILEUX, C. et GOIDIN, E.: Sur les lésions artérielles au cours des traumatismes fermés des membres. Mém. Acad. Chir. *89:* 5 (1963).

GAUTIER, R.; ROULIER, Y.; BOUCHET, G. et COUPPIE: Contusion de l'artère poplitée à la suite d'une luxation du genou en arrière. Désobstruction artérielle. Lyon chir. *55:* 620 (1959).

GIFFORD, R. W.; HINES, E. A., and JANES, J. M.: An analysis and follow-up study of one hundred poppliteal aneurysms. Surgery *33:* 284 (1953).

HORWITZ, T.: Contractura isquémica del miembro inferior. Arch. Surg. *41:* 945 (1940).

HOOVER, N. W.: Lésions de l'artère poplitée associée aux fractures et luxations. Surg. Clin. N. Amer. *41:* 1099 (1961).

HUGHES, C. W.: Acute arterial injuries. Instruct. Course Lecture. Amer. Acad. Orthop. Surg. *12:* (1955).

HUGHES, C. W.: Vascular injuries in the orthopaedic patient. J. Bone Jt Surg. *40A:* 1271 (1958).

JAPAS, L. M. e TRAVERSA, C. H.: El sindrome de Volkmann del miembro inferior. Rev. Ortop. Traumat. lat-amer. *12:* 129 (1967).

JOURDAN, D.: Les ischémies aiguës par fractures de l'extrémité supérieure du tibia; thèse, Montpellier (1959).

KIRKUP, J. R.: Major arterial injury complicating fracture of the femoral shaft. J. Bone Jt Surg. *45B:* 337 (1963).

KIRKUP, J. R.: Lesioni traumatiche dei nervi periferici. 56th Congr. Soc. Ital. Ortop. Traumat., Rome 1971.

LEVEUF, J.: Syndrome de Volkmann. Echec de l'artériectomie. Bull. Mém. Acad. Chir. *61:* 300 (1935).

LUMKIN; LOGAN; CONVES, and HOWARD: Arteriography as an iad in the diagnosis and localisation of acute arterial injuries. Ann. Surg. *147:* 353 (1958).

MAGNANT, J. S.: Plaies vasculaires sèches au cours des fractures diaphysaires des membres. Presse méd. *69:* 594 (1961).

McQUILLAN, W. M. and NOLAN, B.: Ischaemia complicating injury. A report of thirty-seven cases. J. Bone Jt Surg. *50B:* 482 (1968).

MERLE D'AUBIGNÉ, R.; RAMADIER, O. J. *et al.:* Traumatismes anciens. Rachis, Membre inférieur, Paris 1959, p. 391.

MOURGUES, G.; DESCOTES, J.; SISTERON, A. et MOLLARD, P.: Rupture de l'artère poplitée au cours d'une dislocation du genou, Reconstruction artérielle par greffe. Lyon chir. *55:* 600 (1959).

OTTOLENGHI, E. C.: Tratamiento de las lesiones ligamentosas graves de la rodilla. Rev. Ortop. Traumat. lat-amer. *5* (1960).

PERRICONE, G.: Sindrome isquémico di Volkmann dell'artro inferiore. Atti Soc. Emil. Romag. Triv. Ortop. Traumat. *3:* 923 (1958).

PICARD: Fracture de l'épiphyse tibiale supérieure avec troubles vasculaires. Rev. Orthop. *44:* 102 (1958).

PLATT, H.: Traction lesions of the external popliteal nerve. Lancet *1940:* 612.

PORTER, M. F.: Delayed arterial occlusion in limb injuries. J. Bone Jt Surg. *50B:* 138 (1968).

RAFFENSPERGER, J. G. et HINKAMP, J.: Luxation composée du genou avec traumatisme de l'artère poplitée. Arch. Surg. *79:* 799 (1959).

SCAGLIETTI, O.: Le alterazioni dei muscoli nella paralisi di Volkmann. Boll. Mem. Soc. Emil. Chir. *4* (1938).

SCONAMIGLIO: Lesioni vascolari peripheriche di origini traumatica. Arch. Ist. Osp. Santa Corona, *27:* 49 (1962).

SEDDON, H. J.: Volkmann's ischemia in the lower limb. J. Bone Jt Surg. *48B:* 627 (1966).

SEMISCH, W.: Subluxation des Kniegelenkes nach hinten mit Zerreissung der Arteria poplitea. Dtsch. Z. Chir. *243:* 621 (1934).

SINKLER, W. H. and SPENCER, A. D.: Value of peripheral arteriography in acute vascular injury. Arch. Surg. *107:* 228 (1958).

STAHELL, L. T. and FRY, L. R.: Late popliteal false aneurysm complicating distal femoral fracture. J. Trauma *7:* 322 (1967).

STALLWORTH, J. M.; BRADHAM, G. B., and LEE, W. H.: Treatment of peripheral artery aneurysms. Amer. Surg. *27:* 785 (1961).

STEIN, A. H.: Arterial injury in orthopaedic surgery. J. Bone Jt Surg. *38A:* 669 (1956).

STEWART, M. J.; SISK, D., and WALLACE, S. L.: Fractures of the distal third of the femur. J. Bone Jt Surg. *48A:* 784 (1966).

TENEFF, S.: Tecnica chirurgica ortopedica e traumatologica (Soc. Editoria Universo, 1962).

TAYLOR, A. R.; ARDEN, G. P., and RANEY, H. A.: Traumatic dislocation of the knee. J. Bone Jt Surg. *54B:* 96 (1972).

TRAVAINI, E. e VIGNATI, E.: La fisiochinesiergoterapia negli esiti de fratture del piatto tibiale. Minerva Ortop. *18:* 366 (1967).

TRILLAT, A.: Sindrome de Volkmann du membre inférieur. Lyon chir. *49:* 620 (1954).

TOMLINSON, F. B.: A false aneurysm of the popliteal artery due to physical exercise. Report of a case. J. Trauma *7:* 159 (1967).

VITTORI; SAQUET; DUCOURNEAU; AUBRY et THOMAS: Vingt-cinq cas de luxations concomittantes du genou par blast. Mém. Acad. Chir. *8:* 698 (1956).

WATSON-JONES, R.: Fractures y traumatismos articulares; 4th ed. (1952).

WHITE, J.: The results of traction injuries to the common peroneal nerve. J. Bone Jt Surg. *50B:* 346 (1968).

WILSON, W. C.: Occlusion of the main artery and main vein of a limb. Brit. J. Surg. *20:* 393 (1932).

Authors' address: Prof. CARLOS E. OTTOLENGHI and CARLOS H. TRAVERSA, MD, Hospital Italiano, Instituto de Ortopedia y Traumatologia, Potosi 4215, *Buenos Aires* (Argentina)

Reconstr. Surg. Traumat., vol. 14, pp. 136–146 (Karger, Basel 1974)

Longitudinal Fractures of the Patella

Å. Boström

Second Department of Orthopaedic Surgery (Head: Prof. Bertil Stener),
University of Göteborg, Göteborg

Contents

Introduction

Longitudinal fractures of the patella are regarded by some authors as very rare (Dué and Brighenti, 1956; Black and Conners, 1969]. Single cases are reported by many [Lapidus, 1932; Moricca *et al.*, 1961; Teubner and Schreier, 1968; Delic, 1970]. However, Schönbauer [1959] in his series of 578 fractures of the patella reported 12.5 % to be longitudinal fractures and Nummi [1971] in his series of 707 fractures 27.5 %. In the author's series [Boström, 1972] of 422 fractures of the patella 28 % were longitudinal fractures.

Direct violence is held to be the most common cause of longitudinal fractures [Madlener and Paas, 1930; Black and Conners, 1969]. According to Teubner and Schreier [1968] there will be a greater risk of this type of fracture occurring if the appearance of the patella corresponds to types II and III as described by Wiberg [1941]. If the knee is flexed when the injury occurs, the vastus lateralis will produce a lateral dislocation of the fragment [TEUBNER and SCHREIER, 1968]. The dislocation is usually slight, however [DE PALMA, 1954]. The diagnosis may be disregarded, as there are no clinical findings typical of this fracture. The radiograph is unveiling, provided the examination does not only include frontal and lateral views, but also axial projection.

According to SCAPINELLI [1967] longitudinal lateral fractures of the patella and those of the superior lateral angle rarely unite. This he thinks is due to the fact that there is a complete lack of arterial penetration from within the bone to this part of the patella and certainly none inwards from the superior lateral margin. Longitudinal midline fractures – according to the same author – consolidate rapidly because of the absence of the distorting force of the quadriceps and because there is no interruption of the blood supply of the fragments.

Operative treatment of longitudinal lateral fractures with excision of the fragment to prevent pseudarthrosis and, later on, osteoarthrosis is recommended by many [DE PALMA, 1954; O'DONOGHUE, 1958; BÖHLER, 1961; SCAPINELLI, 1967]. Non-operative treatment is recommended by NUMMI [1971], despite the high frequency of pseudarthrosis (14 %), as the late results were hardly affected by non-union.

Primary Series

The series is compiled of patients who, owing to injury of the knee, were radiographically examined in Göteborg during the period 1959 to 1964, and received the diagnosis longitudinal fracture of the patella. Children and adolescents younger than 16 years of age were not included. The only patients included were those with a verified diagnosis of fresh fracture. Those whose diagnosis, fresh or old fracture, was doubtful were excluded, as well as those who had a medial marginal fracture which could have been caused by acute traumatic patellar dislocation [SCHELLER and MÅRTENSON, 1970].

The series includes 92 longitudinal lateral fractures and 25 longitudinal medial, all together 117 fractures; 63 in males (54 %) and 54 in females (46 %). The mean age of the entire series was 47 years; males 38 years and females 57 years. In 63 patients (54 %) the right-sided patella was injured and in 54 (46 %) the left one. No patient had sustained bilateral longitudinal fracture.

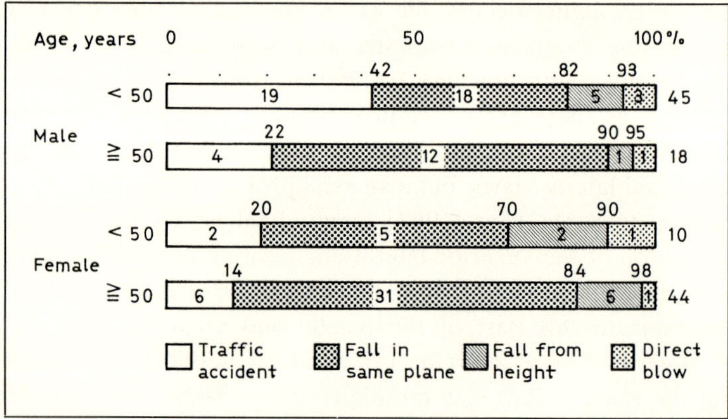

Fig. 1. Mode of injury in longitudinal fracture of the patella in males and females belonging to various age groups. (The figures refer to percentage and number of patients.)

The mode of injury among males and females of various age groups is stated in figure 1. No significant differences in frequency were observed with regard to age and sex. The fractures was caused by other injuries significantly more often than by traffic accidents (p < 0.05).

An open fracture was found in one patient. Concomitant injuries were found in nine patients, two of which sustained bone injuries of the same extremity. Preserved extension capability was recorded in 108 patients (92 %). There was a loss of active function of the quadriceps in four patients and impairment in five. The diastasis between the fragments did not in any case exceed 4 mm. A step in the articular surface of the patella of 1–3 mm was found in eleven patients; in six it exceeded 3 mm.

Non-operative treatment was performed on 112 fractures. As a rule it included immobilization in plaster reaching from the malleoli to the inguen. In some cases the haematoma in the knee was first punctured. An elastic adhesive bandage was regarded as adequate in some cases, whilst in others no treatment was considered necessary.

Operative treatment was performed on five fractures. In two cases the fragment was excised, in one it was nailed with a metal pin and in two the fragment was fastened with silk sutures.

The approximate median period of immobilization in plaster after non-surgical as well as surgical treatment was three weeks.

The median period of sick-leave was less than two months. After that time 68 % were discharged as restored.

Table I. Estimation of subjectively experienced impairment of function

Subjectively experienced impairment of function	Age, years	
	≥ 60	< 60
Feeling of unsteadiness or weakness	1	2
Limping		
Following exertions	0	1
Always	1	2
Support		
Only outdoors	1	1
Always	2	2
Walking distance		
Impaired (< 5 km)	2	2
Severely impaired (< 1 km)	4	4
Walking up and down stairs		
Slowly but with alternating steps	1	1
Mounting stairs with healthy leg first and descending stairs with injured leg first	2	2
Running, impaired	0	2
Sports, impaired	0	2
Maximal score	10	16

Follow-Up Study

The follow-up study included 88 subjects, constituting 91 % of those alive at the time of the investigation. Of these, 66 subjects had sustained a longitudinal lateral fracture of the patella and 22 a longitudinal medial fracture. The time of observation varied from 5 to 12 years. The mean time of observation was nine years. Of the 88 subjects, 71 were thoroughly examined according to the method mentioned below. A further four subjects, who were elderly, were examined in their homes and the remaining 13 answered questionnaires, but were not examined. The mean age of the subjects followed up was 52 years, i. e. for 49 males 45 years and for 39 females 60 years.

Methods

The nature and degree of pain and the subjectively experienced impairment of function was assessed on the basis of verbal and/or written questioning. Ache and pain were classified according to the following: (1) Temporary ache, e. g. with atmospheric changes or in kneeling posture. (2) Ache when starting to walk or in connection with a lengthy position, e. g. in a squatting posture. (3) Ache in connection with exertions. (4) Ache caused by all activities. (5) Pain at rest.

In analyzing the impairment of function consideration was taken to the age of the subject. An age limit of 60 years was selected and the functions included were scored (table I).

At the clinical examination, walking on a level surface as well as the capability of mounting and descending stairs were assessed. Extension defect and range of mobility of the knee joints were measured with an angle gauge. The maximal circumference of the calf, the circumference on a level with the patella, and the circumference of the thigh, 15 cm proximally to the medial interarticular space, were measured on both legs.

The force of the extensor muscles was measured in a special chair designed by HÖÖK and TORNVALL [1969] and equipped with a strain gauge dynamometer for measuring isometric power of muscles. The knee was flexed through 90°. The maximal force was recorded – after several attempts, the last value obtained being lower than the highest – and a percentage of the reduction of force was calculated on the force of the uninjured leg.

Radiographs were taken of both knee joints including frontal, lateral and axial projections. For loading the patellofemoral joint while the axial projection was taken, the subjects was standing with the patella to be examined resting against a support, mounted on a special examining stand, and with the knee in a semi-flexed position [AHLBÄCK, 1968].

Appraisal of the consolidation of the fracture, fibrous union and pseudarthrosis was included in the radiographic analysis, as well as enlargement of the patella and formation and development of osteoarthrosis. For the estimation of osteo-arthrosis the most important factors were changes of the structure – deformation of articular surfaces, presence of cysts, and subchondral sclerosis – and a reduced joint space. The presence of osteophytes was not sufficient evidence for osteoarthrosis to be diagnosed. Osteoarthrosis was recorded and classified according to KELLGREN and LAWRENCE [1957] and KELLGREN [1963].

Results

The pain in the injured knee was considered as slight if it occurred in connection with kneeling or atmospheric changes, and as moderate if it occurred when starting to walk and as the result of a lengthy squatting posture or during exertions. The pain was regarded as severe if it persisted at rest and/or in all activities. It was found that 51 subjects (58 %)

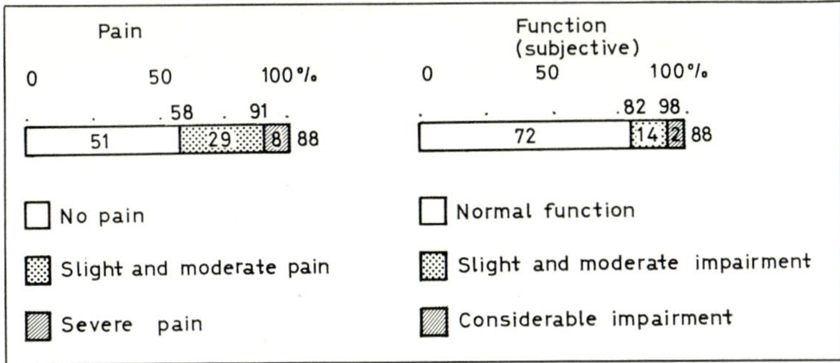

Fig. 2. Subjective symptoms after longitudinal fracture of the patella.

had no pain and 17 (20 %) had slight pain. Moderate pain was noted in 12 (13 %) and severe in 8 (9 %) subjects (fig. 2).

The subjectively experienced impairment of function was considered slight if the corresponding score did not exceed 2 points. The impairment of function was moderate if the score exceeded 2 but not 4 and 6 points, respectively. If the score was higher the impairment of function was classified as considerable. No abnormality of the function was stated by 72 subjects (82 %). Slight impairment of function was found in 7 (8 %), moderate in 7 (8 %) and considerable in 2 (2 %) subjects (fig. 2).

The range of mobility of the injured knee was considered as normal if there was no deficiency of extension and if the knee could be flexed to at least 120°. It was considered as restricted if there was a deficiency of extension and/or the bending capacity to a flexed position of less than 120° could be measured. The restriction was regarded as moderate if the deficiency of extension was 10° or less and/or the bending capacity could be measured to a flexed position of less than 120° but more than 90°. It was regarded as considerable if the deficiency of extension exceded 10° and/or the bending capacity to a flexed position of 90° or less could be measured. The range of mobility of the injured knee was normal in 73 subjects (97 %). Moderate restriction was recorded in 2 subjects (3 %) and considerable in none (table II).

The circumference of the thighs was regarded as equal if the difference in the values measured was nil or less than 1 cm. If the circumference of the thigh was reduced by at least 1 cm, atrophy of the quadriceps musculature was assumed. Atrophy was assessed as moderate if the reduction was less than 2 cm, and considerable if the reduction was at

Table II. Objective signs after longitudinal fracture of the patella

	Normal		Restricted/reduced			
			moderately		considerably	
	number	percent	number	percent	number	percent
Range of mobility	73	97	2	3	0	0
Circumference of the thigh	63	84	10	13	2	3
Extension force at the knee	55	73	17	23	3	4

least 2 cm. The circumference of the thighs was equal in 63 subjects (84 %). Atrophy of the injured side was moderate in 10 (13 %) and considerable in 2 (3 %) (table II).

The extension force of the knees was regarded as equal if the same value, including a decrease or increase of 10 %, was obtained for both sides. The extension force of the injured side was considered to be reduced if the reduction was more than 10 %. The reduction of force was classified as moderate if the reduction was less than 30 %, and considerable if the reduction was at least 30 %. Equal force was measured in 55 subjects (73 %). Moderate reduction of force was noted in 17 (23 %) and considerable in 3 (4 %) subjects (table II).

The fracture had united in 56 subjects (79 %). Fibrous union was established in 12 subjects (17 %) and pseudarthrosis in 3 (4 %) (fig. 3). The fact that they had pseudarthrosis was unknown to them.

A step in the articular surface of the patella of 1 mm or more was established in 8 subjects (11 %).

Enlargement of the patella was considered to exist if an increase of width of at least 1/2 cm could be measured on the radiograph. 14 (20 %) had enlargement of the patella of the injured side.

Osteoarthrotic changes in the injured patellofemoral joint were observed in 8 subjects (11 %). However, as radiographs were taken of both the knees and also were available from the time of injury, it was possible to establish, whether the osteoarthrotic changes had become increased in comparison with the opposite side and with the time of injury. Progressive osteoarthrosis was diagnosed in only 4 subjects (6 %), none of whom having osteoarthrosis in the femorotibial joint of the injured side.

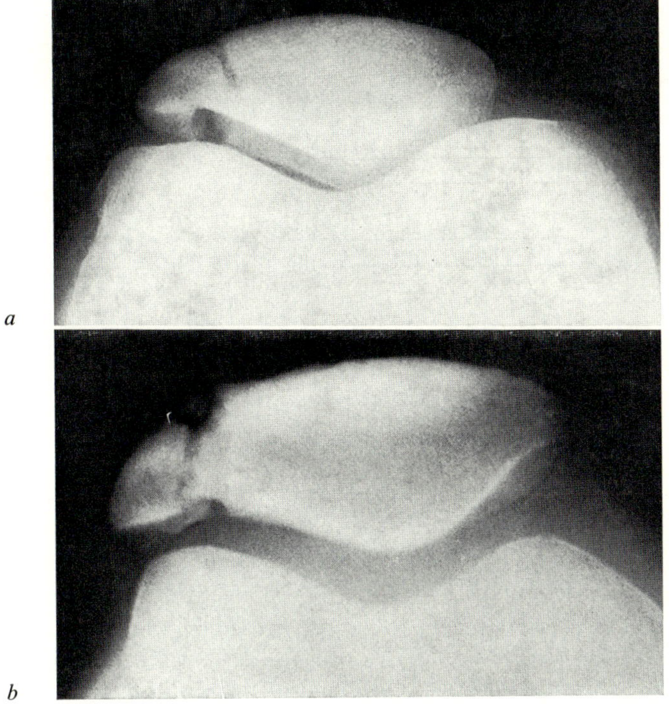

Fig. 3. Longitudinal fracture of the patella *(a)*, treated with immobilization in plaster. Fibrous union six years later *(b)*. (The late result was good [BOSTRÖM, 1972)].

Osteoarthrosis – irrespective of the genesis – depended on the age of the subjects at the follow-up examination and was significantly more often found in those over 60 years of age. Osteoarthrosis of the knee occurred twice as often in females as in males. There was no increase in the frequency of osteoarthrosis of the patellofemoral joint because of fibrous union, pseudarthrosis and enlargement of the patella. The frequency of osteoarthrosis was insignificantly higher in those with a step in the articular surface of the patella of 1 mm or more as compared with the other series.

The result was considered *excellent* if the subject was free from discomfort without pain or subjectively experienced impairment of function, with a normal range of mobility of the knee-joint, and with equal force in the extensor apparatus of both knees. The result was considered *poor*

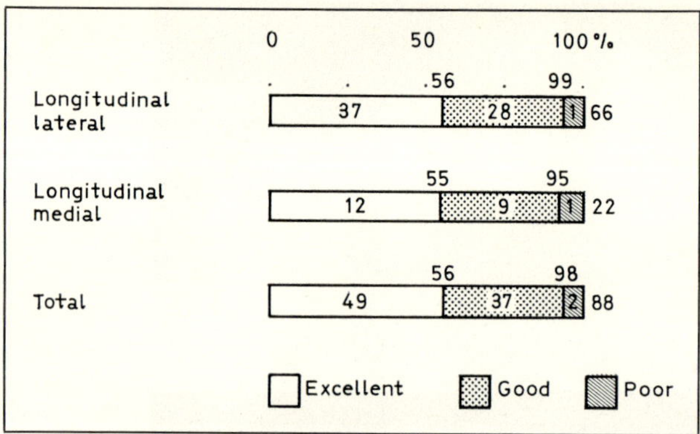

Fig. 4. Late results after longitudinal fractures of the patella.

if the injury alone could be assumed to be the cause of pain at rest and/or pain during all kinds of activity. Furthermore, the result was regarded as poor if the injury alone could be assumed to be the cause of at least two of the following three symptoms and signs: (1) Subjectively experienced impairment of function corresponding to a score exceeding 4 and 6 points, respectively. (2) Deficiency of extension exceeding 10° and/or bending capacity to a flexed position of 90° or less. (3) Reduction of force of the extensor apparatus of the knee exceeding 30 % of the force of the un-injured knee.

In all the other cases the result was considered *good*. Subjects with a good result formed a heterogenous group. In this group were included, in addition to those with a good result on account of the injury, also those with a poor result that was not ascribable to the injury but instead probably caused by another disease, e. g. osteoarthrosis not being connected with the injury. If it had been possible in these cases to assess the real result of the injury, one or other of the subjects might have been referred either to the group excellent or to the group poor results.

Excellent results were achieved in 49 (56 %) and good results in 37 subjects (42 %). The results were poor in 2 (2 %) subjects (fig. 4). The one was a male of 57 years of age with a large medial fragment, which was excised. Possibly it had been better to restore the normal anatomy with one or two screws. The other was a male of 61 years of age who sustained a lateral fracture with 2–3 mm diastasis between the fragments. He developed a painful osteoarthrosis in the injured patellofemoral joint and received a disablement pension.

Discussion

Longitudinal fracture of the patella is – contrary to the opinion held in most earlier reports – a common type of patellar fracture. As the continuity of the extensor apparatus of the knee joint is not interrupted, its diagnosis can be missed. Many times the fracture is unveiled only by a thorough radiographic examination, including axial projection. The fracture may result from different modes of injury.

Subjective symptoms occur to a considerable extent after longitudinal patellar fracture. As the period of observation in this report was nine years and the mean age at the follow-up examination was 52 years, it is necessary to bear in mind that there may be other reasons for the joint discomfort than the sequelae of patellar fracture. Restricted range of mobility, atrophy of the quadriceps muscle and reduced extensor force of the knees may also be found irrespective of the injury. Many authors have pointed out that osteoarthrosis may set in after a joint lesion. In this investigation, it was possible to distinguish between osteoarthrosis ascribable to the injury and osteoarthrosis which could depend on other circumstances. A rather high frequency of osteoarthrosis unrelated to the injury could be expected, as the higher age groups included many females [HERNBORG, 1969]. Without doubt, however, osteoarthrosis may develop as a direct result of the injury.

Excellent and good results after longitudinal fracture of the patella were achieved to a large extent, a fact experienced also by NUMMI [1971]. In no case of fibrous union and pseudarthrosis were the late results poor. This investigations does not support the opinion held, for instance, by DE PALMA [1954] that longitudinal lateral fractures should be treated surgically in order to avoid future discomfort. However, opeative treatment with excision of the fragment may be justified exceptionally, e. g. in open fractures.

Summary

Longitudinal fracture of the patella is a common type of patellar fracture. In a series of 422 fractures of the patella 117 (28 %) were longitudinal. The radiograph is revealing, provided the examination includes axial projection. Non-operative treatment with immobilization in plaster for three weeks is sufficient. Despite fibrous union and pseudarthrosis the late result is good. In this series excellent and good results were obtained in 98 % after a mean time of observation of nine years.

References

Ahlbäck, S.: Osteoarthrosis of the knee. A radiographic investigation; thesis. Acta radiol., Stockh. Suppl. 277 (1968).

Black, J. K. and Conners, J. J.: Vertical fractures of the patella. Sth. med. J. *62:* 76–77 (1969).

Boström, Å.: Fracture of the patella. A study of 422 patellar fractures; thesis. Acta orthop. scand. Suppl. 143 (1972).

Böhler, J.: Behandlung der Kniescheibenbrüche. Osteosynthese, Teilexstirpation, Exstirpation. Dtsch. med. Wschr. *86:* 1209–1212 (1961).

Delic, M.: Rezesione nella frattura marginale della rotula. Minerva ortop. *21:* 266–269 (1970).

Dué, G. e Brighenti, G. M.: Sulla frattura verticale della rotula. Arch. Ortop., Milano *69:* 373–387 (1956).

Hernborg, J.: Knäledsarthrosens naturalhistoria (Föredrag vid Medicinsk Riksstämma, Stockholm 1969).

Höök, O. and Tornvall, G.: Apparatus and method for determination of isometric muscle strength in man. Scand. J. Rehab. Med. *1:* 139–142 (1969).

Kellgren, J. H. and Lawrence, J. S.: Radiological assessment of osteo-arthrosis. Ann. rheum. Dis. *16:* 494–502 (1957).

Kellgren, J. H.: The epidemiology of chronic rheumatism. Atlas of standard radiographs of arthritis (Blackwell, Oxford 1963).

Lapidus, P. W.: Longitudinal fractures of the patella. J. Bone Jt Surg. *14A:* 351–379 (1932).

Madlener, J. M. und Paas, H. R.: Über Patellarfrakturen und ihre Folgezustände, unter besonderer Berücksichtigung der Arthritis deformans. Arch. klin. Chir. *156:* 445–462 (1930).

Moricca, F.; Gili, G. e Donadio, F.: Frattura verticale della rotula. Minerva ortop. *12:* 388–390 (1961).

Nummi, J.: Fracture of the patella. A clinical study of 707 patellar fractures; thesis. Ann. Chir. Gynaec. Fenn. Suppl. 179 (1971).

O'Donoghue, D. H.: Treatment of fractures of the patella. Nw. Med., Seattle *57:* 1592–1600 (1958).

Palma, A. F. de: Diseases of the knee (Lippincott, Philadelphia 1954).

Scapinelli, R.: Blood supply of the human patella. Its relation to ischaemic necrosis after fracture. J. Bone Jt Surg. *49B:* 563–570 (1967).

Scheller, S. and Mårtenson, L.: Traumatisk patellarluxation. Föredrag vid Nordisk Ortopedisk Förenings 35. kongress, Århus 1970.

Schönbauer, H. R.: Brüche der Kniescheibe. Ergebn. Chir. Orthop. *42:* 56–79 (1959).

Teubner, E. und Schreier, G.: Klinik und Therapie der Patellalängsfrakturen (Bericht über 10 Fälle). Mschr. Unfallheilk. *71:* 426–438 (1968).

Wiberg, G.: Roentgenographic and anatomic studies on the femoropatellar joint. Acta orthop. scand. *12:* 319–410 (1941).

Author's address: Dr. Åke Boström, Department of Orthopaedic Surgery II, University of Göteborg, *Göteborg* (Sweden)

Reconstr. Surg. Traumat., vol. 14, pp. 147–152 (Karger, Basel 1974)

The Use of Ultrasonic Instrumentation
for the Transection and Uniting of Bone Tissue
in Orthopaedic Surgery

M. V. VOLKOV and I. S. SHEPELEVA

Priorov Central Institute for Traumatology and Orthopaedics
(Director: Prof. M. V. VOLKOV), Moscow

Various instruments such as saws, chisels, osteotomes and cutters are generally used for transecting biological tissues – particularly bone. In addition, some physical effort is necessary and there is a certain time loss involved. These techniques can be regarded as relatively coarse and do not correspond to the possibilities of modern technology. They often result in cracking and splintering of the bone and irregularities of the cut surface. Such complications can occur even in the hands of experienced surgeons who are well acquainted with the instruments. Many methods involve hammering or jarring of the bone, for example the skull. These can lead to unfavourable reactions on the part of the patient which must be ascribed to technical imperfections.

The use of Dalgren punches is complicated. The punches become blocked and have to be cleaned frequently during the operation. Gigli saws as used for operations on the skull are not only dangerous but impractical. When used for other parts of the body, these saws require the wide separation of the handles. This is not without problems in small, deep operative wounds. The rotation or vibration saws cause undesired heating of the bone and spread bone particles into the surroundings.

Excellent cooperation between our engineers and orthopaedic surgeons has led to the development of a method for the transection of biological tissue using ultrasonic instruments.

Osteotomy is most frequently employed for the correction of bone deformities and defective positions of the joints. Until very recently it was performed with conventional instruments resulting in the disadvantages mentioned above.

In 1969 VOLKOV used ultrasonic instruments for the transection and

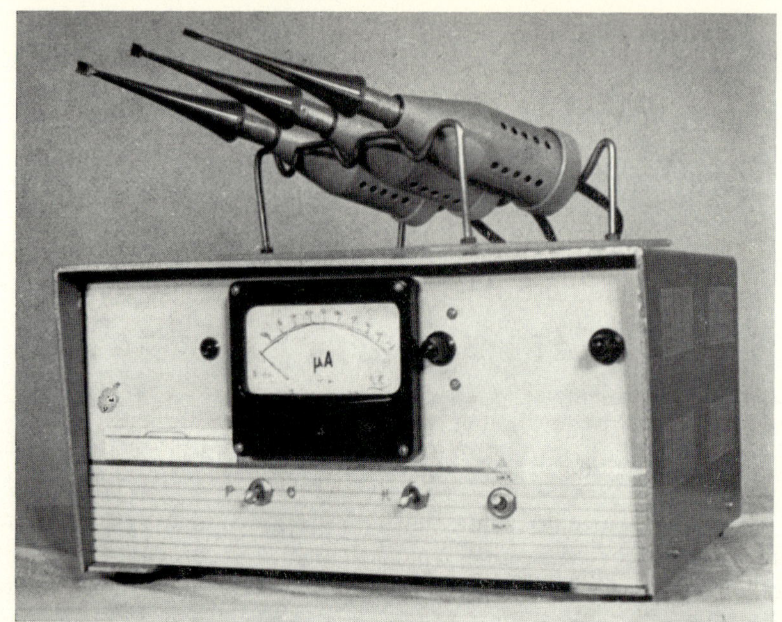

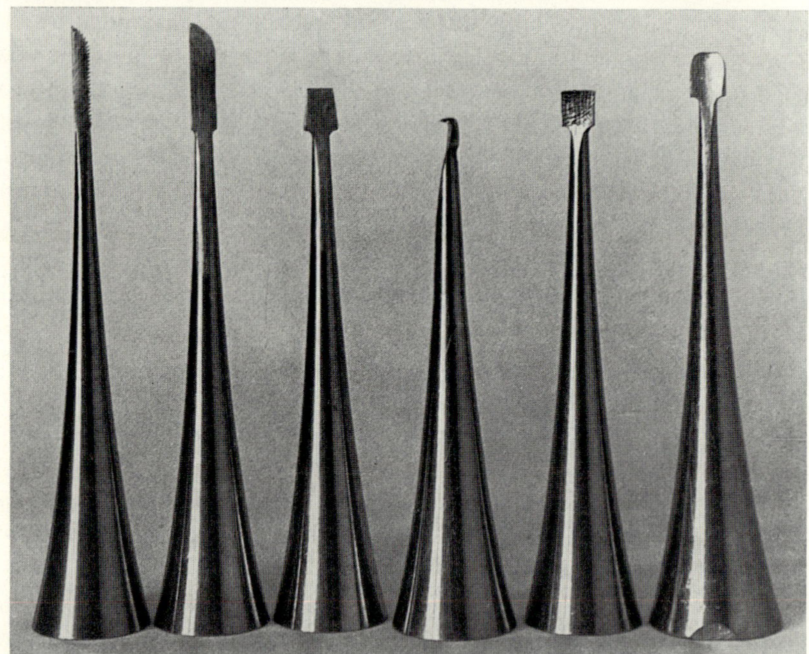

Fig. 1. The URSK-7N apparatus.
Fig. 2. A set of exchangeable ultrasound conducting instruments.

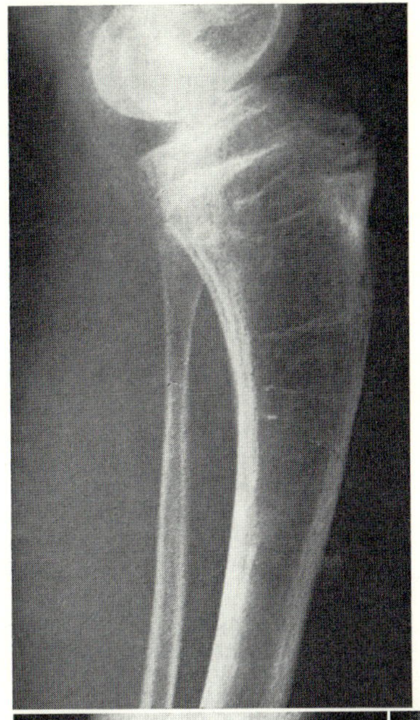

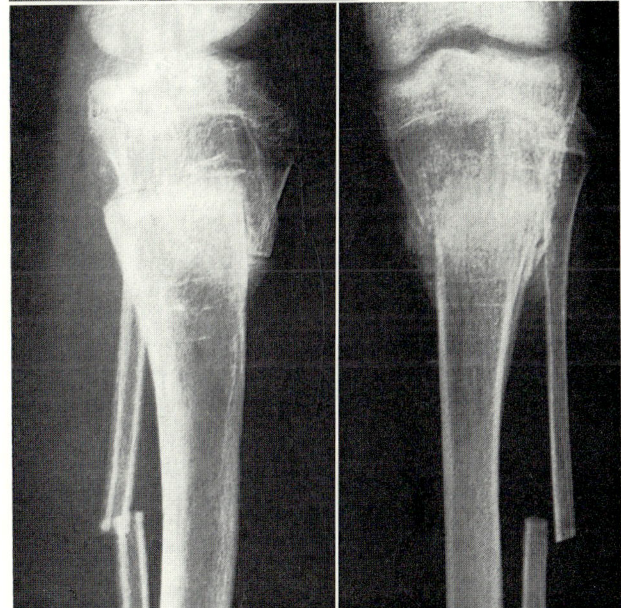

Fig. 3. Severe deformity of the right tibia in a 15-year-old girl (U. R.).

Fig. 4a, b. Deformity in the right tibia of patient U. R. due to osteogenosis imperfecta.

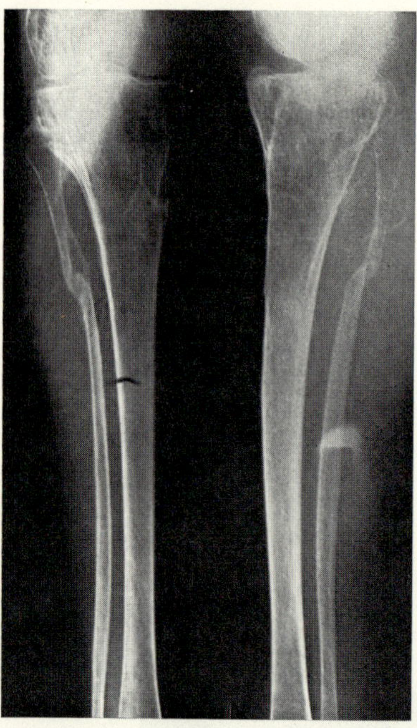

Fig. 5. Final result of correction in patient U. R.

rejoining of bone tissue in orthopaedics for the first time. The development of an ultrasonic instrumentation in surgery started in 1964 at first on an experimental basis and then in traumatology (G. A. NIKOLAJEV, V. A. POLJAKOV, V. J. LOSHJILOV and G. G. TCHEMJANOV).

We use the apparatus (URSK-7N (fig. 1), with a set of exchangeable ultrasound conducting instruments (fig. 2) for transection, rejoining and sawing of biological tissue. The wave amplitude is not below 50 mk and the frequency is 25–30 kHz. The temperature during rejoining of the bone does not exceed 70–80 °C and the duration of such temperatures is limited to a few seconds (V. O. LEONITCHEV, 1971).

We have performed various types of osteotomies with the help of ultrasound including transverse, straight, inclined and Z-shaped osteotomies and even those involving a geometrical figure. Certain types of osteotomy also allow lengthening of the bone.

The following case is cited as an illustration: The patient, U. R., was a 15-year-old girl (fig. 3). A correction osteotomy followed by osteosynthesis was performed with the help of ultrasonic apparatus on 26. 12. 1969 because of severe deformity of the right tibia due to osteogenesis imperfecta (fig. 4a, b). Figure 5 shows the final result of the correction.

Our experiences with bone transection in various types of deformities includes 311 cases. With the help of ultrasonic saws, it is possible to work from a small, approximately 2-cm incision. Thus, it is possible to cut off juvenile exostoses at their base without damage to the soft tissue.

The principle of joining bones together involves the implantation of auto-, homo- or heterografts in the form of small fragments between the bones or in the bone defect, and soaking them with an additional material. Under the influence of ultrasonic waves, complex physico-chemical processes result in a conglomerate of the bone fragments which bind the bones firmly together. Ethyl α-cyanacrylate (Cyacryn) is used in addition which acts as a glue, binding the bone chips to the recipient bone. The processes of bone transformation, incorporation and osteogenesis follow normally. Rejoining of bone with ultrasound instrumentation has been attempted in 207 cases including osteotomy in the desired position, obtaining a reliable bridge between homografts and recipient bone and filling up postoperative defects after resection. Experimental results and clinical experience have shown that it is advantageous when the artificial callus is restricted to a third of the bone circumference so that two thirds are left for the development of the natural bone callus.

No disadvantages have been observed in the use of ultrasound instrumentation in children's orthopaedics for cases with marked osteoporisis (osteogenesis imperfecta, fibrous osteodysplasia, morbus Blount, etc.), whereas normal mechanical tools damage the bone. One of the greatest advantages of ultrasonic saws is the possibility of approaching the bone through a very small incision even in cases of longitudinal separation of the cortex. This is desirable when performing decortication, Z-shaped lengthening osteotomies, inclined osteotomies and even for the economical resection of bone tumours in the region of healthy bone.

Conclusions

1. Ultasonic instrumentation considerably simplifies orthopaedic operations including the removal of bone tumours.

2. The ultrasonic consolidation of bone guarantees a rapid and firm union between the bone fragments. The artificial callus resorbs without disturbing the regenerative processes of the bone which take place at the normal time.

Authors' address: Prof. M. V. VOLKOV and Dr. I. S. SHEPELEVA, Priorov Central Institute for Traumatology and Orthopaedics, Ul. Priorova 10, *Moscow A-299* (USSR)

Editorial Note

It is of importance and interest to deal with psychological problems in patients belonging to our speciality – orthopaedic and reconstruction surgery as well as traumatology. These two articles are the first ones of a series we hope to continue.

Starting with the relation parents/child and child/parents, we shall try to submit to our readers articles on the psychology of injured and deformed patients, as far as this knowledge may be of use in taking therapeutic decisions.

GEORGE CHAPCHAL

Reconstr. Surg. Traumat., vol. 14, pp. 154–156 (Karger, Basel 1974)

The Relationship of Parents after the Birth of a Child with a Congenital Defect

S. Rafalovich

The family balance is created by common wishes, expectations and hopes. The family grows by the addition of children. The expectations, plans and the birth of a healthy child, create the family image. The relations between the parents has a past and a present – this fact enables us to make a guess for future relations.

After the expectation of a healthy child, the disappointment at the birth of a child with a defect spoils the family image. The situation thus created leads us to expect a change in parental relations.

In 39 clinical observations, this new situation did not change the parental relations which existed before the birth of this child. If the relations have been based on mutual support, the same situation will prevail and the opposite is also true. If there were disagreements between the parents before the birth, the parents will project them onto che child with the defect.

This situation can be graphically demonstrated:

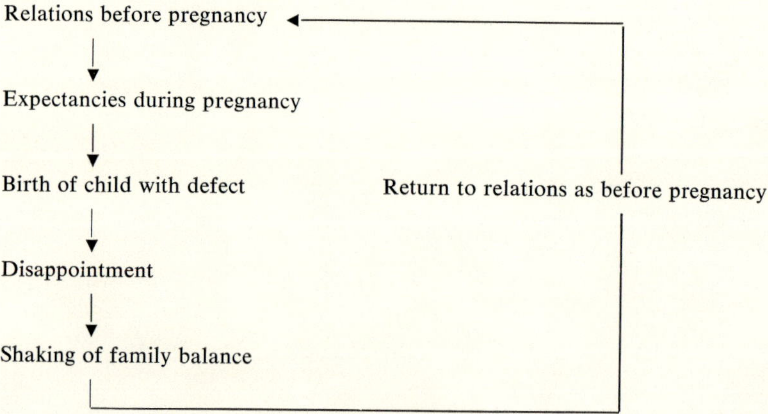

The weak link in this graphically demonstrated sequence is the 'disappointment'. This step is turned into the center of the whole problem. Here starts our intervention in helping the parents to express their feelings openly. This should bring into the focus the real relations between the parents and their relations to the defective child.

For example, the parents of M. L. were married by civil marriage (not existing in our Jewish law); the mother refused an abortion, and the father objected to the marriage. For that reason, they travelled to England and were married in front of a lawyer, pointing out that this is not a real planned marriage. After the birth of the child with loss of left forearm and hand, the father blamed the mother for the imposed marriage. The father focused all his attention towards the defect of the child, not realizing that his problem is the acceptance of the mother of the child, his own wife.

Another example is the parents of G. D. The mother went to university, the father has primary school education only. The mother wishes additional children, while the father blames himself for his weakness, having accepted her will with such a disastrous result. With the birth of the child, one parent blamed the family of the other for some genetic deficiency. All this reflects only the fact that disagreement between the two parents existed before the birth of the child.

In the group of 39 parents there is no divorce case, but one couple separated before it was known to them that the mother was pregnant. Of the same group, in 17 families the defective child is over 10 years of age, while in the remaining 22 families, the age of the defective child is below 5 years. In the first group of families the additional children prove that the family ties are strongly developed, while in the second group, the time of observation is too short to draw any conclusions.

Referring to my scheme of sequences, it is worthwhile mentioning that in the stage of the most severe crisis, there is no separation of the parents. On the contrary, the relations seem to improve under the pressure of the responsibility, as in the previously mentioned case of M. L. where we doubt if the husband would have continued the family relation without his feelings towards the child.

The observation of 39 families demonstrates different reactions by the parents of a defective child. Families in which disagreements existed before the birth are disregarded. Their problems are reflected upon the child. The contrary is true in families with close relations, the defective child increases the mutual support of the parents.

Summary

The birth of a defective child spoils the family image, a fact which leads us to expect a change in parental relations. In 39 clinical observations, we found that this new situation did not change parental relations. After the disappointment with a birth of such a child, the relations return to be those which existed before the birth. If the relations have been based on mutual support, the same situation will prevail, and if there were disagreements before, the parents will project them onto the child with the defect.

References

1   HOEK, S.: Some problems of mothers of handicapped children. Megamot *12:* 146–153 (1962).
2   JORDAN, T. E.: Physical disability in children and family adjustment. Rehabilitation Lit. *24:* 330–336 (1962).

Author's address: Dr. S. RAFALOVICH, BA, Tel Hashomer Hospital, *Tel-Aviv* (Israel)

Reconstr. Surg. Traumat., vol. 14, pp. 157–160 (Karger, Basel 1974)

Guilt Feelings in Parents of Children with Congenital Defects

S. GUR

The guilt feelings of parents of children with congenital defects play an important part in their reaction after the birth. In this paper we concentrate mostly on the mother, as we see in her the central figure in this phase of development. The attitude of the mother determines her reaction to the physical and emotional needs of the child. These reactions are important for the child to perceive himself and his surroundings. It determines to a great extent the strength of the child's ego.

To be a mother implies finding gratification in taking care of her child. In return, the child feels accepted. The birth of a child with a defect creates feelings of guilt, sorrow, doubts and anxiety in the mother.

There is a belief that the mother bears all the responsibility for a normal pregnancy. Any damage to the new born creates in her guilt feelings. If these feelings are not resolved, they may develop into a chronic state which can effect the mother-child relationship. This can be expressed in different ways. The child can identify himself with the feelings of his mother, like guilt, fear and aggressiveness. The mother is never satisfied with the achievments of the child, she criticizes negatively his activities and demands performances above his capacity.

Overconciousness of the mother towards the education of her child creates hypersensitivity in the child's mind and results in guilt feelings in the child, he feels concern that anything he does is wrong.

An example that illustrates this is as follows:

M. Z.: Terminal transverse meromelia of fingers, age 18, child of a family that lives on welfare. The father is hospitalized in a mental hospital, the mother has strong guilt feelings, she offered her fingers to be transplanted to M. Z. M. Z. expresses guilt which results in feeling inferior.

Motherhood demands to be free of internal conflicts or to be able to cope with them. The mother who gives birth to a child with a defect is torn between her inner conflicts and her immediate responsibility towards the child. She has not enough emotional energy to meet the child's needs.

Two examples that reflect this situation:

G. N.: Longitudinal proximal meromelia of radius and 3 fingers. The first born, 2 weeks old. The parents are still under the influence of the tragic event. The mother continues to cry, and the father escapes daily confrontation. The mother does not change the baby's clothes in order to avoid seeing the defect. The family tries to diminish the tragedy by suppressing the appropriate reactions of the mother, her crying, and expressing her callous feelings.

B. A.: Longitudinal proximal meromelia of radius and 3 fingers, 6 months old, third child. This time the pregnancy was unwanted by the mother and wanted by the father. He has guilt feelings. The parent's reactions are mitigated by the fact that their previous children are normal.

The most shattering example of inadequacy to face responsibility as parents are as follows:

K. A.: Terminal defect of both feet with bowing of tibia, terminal defect of 3 fingers and metacarpals of the left hand, 6-month-old, first child. In first 2 months the mother refused to see the child. The parents refuse to take him home. He is in a maternity home. The mother is preoccupied with her inner conflicts.

Another example is as follows:

P. O.: Terminal defects of both hands and fingers, terminal defect of both feet, 1-year-old, second child. The first child is without defects. The same situation occurred here, but this child is in a foster family where the foster mother is developing motherly feelings towards the child.

Some parents, particularly mothers, do not stop to crying in order to express their dispair and their wish to die. This fits into Freud's theory of mourning and melancholia. To come to grips with the mourning is a long and slow process. 21 out of 39 mothers that are included in this study are still within this state of mind even after a long period of time. This is expressed by repeated time consuming telling of their sad stories. Slowly and gradually they express their intensive feelings connected with a distraction from a rosy dream.

Similar and confused intensions charactizes the doctor and nurses at the delivery of the child. They try to defer personal decisions and wish to delay every care connected with the physical defect. They mostly do not realize that the most urgent problems are the parents and the psychological state of their minds.

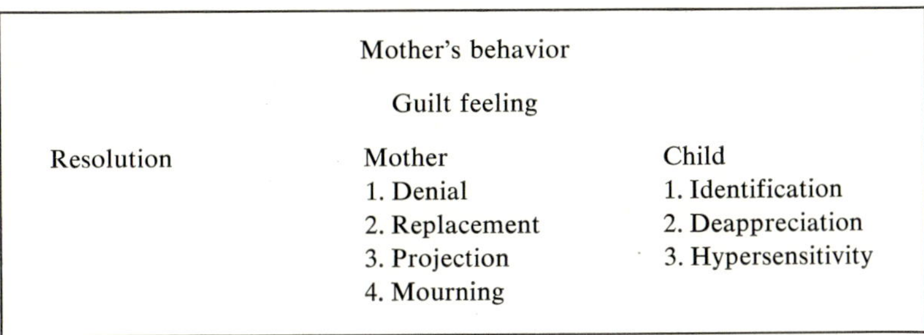

Fig. 1. Diagram of mother's behavior after giving birth to a child with a defect.

We learned from our experience that the earlier we play a part in dealing with the parents, the clearer the situation will be. Our team: the orthopedist, the psychologist and the social worker, approach the parents with immediate attention. We try to evaluate the problems and start to meet their medical, economic and socio-psychological needs. Our immediate task is to provide them with a perceptive situation where they can feel free to express their fears, anxieties and guilt feelings.

We believe that as long as the mother regards herself as the cause of the defect, she will not be able to give the attention and the protection the child needs.

If the mother finds the courage and power to approach her traumatic experience, only then will she make peace with herself and will be able to bring up her child.

Summary

In the birth of a child with a defect, the mother's behavior is dominated by guilt feelings. These feelings can be resolved or they may increase the inner conflicts of the mother in many ways. They can be transferred to the child, who may develop similar reactions.

Proper attention is given to the importance of the reactions of the medical and nursing attendents during the period after the birth of the child.

We conclude that our task is to help the mother and father to resolve their guilt feelings, so as to enable them to meet the child's needs for growth.

References

1 DEUTSCH, M.: Psychology of women, vol. II, p. 17 (Grune & Stratton, New York 1945).
2 FREUD, S.: Mourning and melancholia, collected papers, vol. VIII, pp. 152–170 (1959).
3 HOEK, S.: Some problems of mothers of handicaped children, vol. 12, pp. 147–153 (Megamot 1962).
4 JORDEN, F.: Physical disability in children and family adjustment. Rehabilitation Lit. *24:* 330–336 (1963).
5 POWER, A. *et al.:* Mother-child relationship in rehabilitation of the physical disabled. Social Casework *32:* 261–265 (1951).

Author's address: Dr. S. GUR, MSc, Rehabilitation Psychologist, Tel Hashomer Hospital, *Tel-Aviv* (Israel)